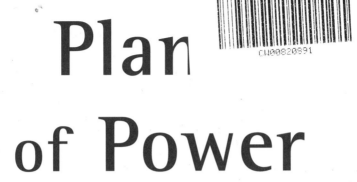

Plan
of Power

Native American Ceremony
and the
Use of Sacred Plants

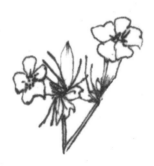

Alfred Savinelli

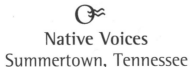

Native Voices
Summertown, Tennessee

© 2002 Alfred Savinelli

Illustrations by Dove Abbot

Cover design by Warren Jefferson

Interior design by Jerry Hutchens

Native Voices

A division of Book Publishing Company
P. O. Box 99
Summertown, TN 38483

(888) 260-8458
www.bookpubco.com

12 11   8 7 6 5

ISBN: 1-57067-130-3
978-1-57067-130-2
Printed in Canada by Transcontinental

Savinelli, Alfred, 1953-
  Plants of power : Native American ceremony and the use of sacred plants / Alfred Savinelli.
     p. cm.
Includes bibliographical references and index.
  ISBN 1-57067-130-3
  1. Indians of North America--Rites and ceremonies. 2. Indians of North America--Ethnobotany. 3. Indian cosmology--North America. 4. Plants--North America--Religious aspects. 5. Medicinal plants--North America. 6. Aromatic plants--North America. I. Title.
  E98.R53 S28 2002
  299'.74--dc21

                         2002004296

The Book Publishing Co. is a member of Green Press Initiative. We elected to print this title on paper with 100% postconsumer recycled content and processed chlorine free, which saved the following natural resources:

9 trees	392 lbs of solid waste
3,059 gallons of water	735 lbs of greenhouse gases
6 million BTUs	

green
press
INITIATIVE

For more information visit: www.greenpressinitiative.org.
Savings calculations thanks to the Environmental Defense Paper Calculator at www.papercalculator.org

For your favorite Native American books and tapes visit
www.nativevoices.com

Table of Contents

Part II

The Plants

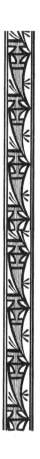

Beseeching the breath of the divine one,
      His life-giving breath,
      His breath of old age,
      His breath of waters,
      His breath of seeds,
      His breath of riches,
      His breath of fecundity,
      His breath of power,
      His breath of strong spirit,
      His breath of all good fortune
          whatsoever,
Asking for his breath
And into my warm body drawing his breath,
I add to your breath
That happily you may always live.

                   Zuni

Introduction

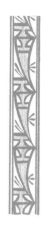

This book is for people who seek to connect more fully with mystery, with the nonhuman world of plants, animals and spirit. Our contemporary society has become too human centered and materialistic. This separates us from each other and our source. We forget the spiritual nature that lives within and behind all forms. We have attached ourselves to certain beliefs about the way things are, and these beliefs often imprison us.

To bring our lives back into alignment with the cosmos, to reconnect with the source that deeply feeds us, to remember that life is but a dream and we are, collectively, its dreamers requires vigilance. We must keep remembering. Tribal peoples used ritual to remember. Historically, the ritual was a dynamic act harkening back to a spiritual event that took the people by surprise and brought them close together

Remake ordinary time and space into sacred time and space.

in collective awe before a beautiful manifestation of spirit. The people created rituals to enact these events. Native American Indian literature often describes miracles in which the Great Spirit sent messages to instruct the people in appropriate ritual forms. The priests of the tribes were seized with inspiration and received vision. This was witnessed by others who then enacted the proscribed rites for their people and future generations.

We invite spirit into our homes and workplaces.

How do we as modern peoples bring ritual back into our daily lives? First, we remake ordinary time and space into sacred time and space by recognizing the spiritual aspect that lives within and behind all forms and structures that we take for granted. All doors are portals; all hallways are passageways; all automobiles are symbols of transit into the unknown. When we enhance seemingly ordinary things and daily routines with offerings of smoke and prayer, we invite spirit into our homes and workplaces.

Native American peoples have long known the special attributes or personalities of sacred plants. Living close to the earth in communion and collaboration with plants and animals, the people recognize plant's special properties. Current research, based in western scientific method, has often corroborated ancient wisdom about the spiritual, medicinal properties of plants; forty to fifty percent of western pharmaceuticals were originally derived from compounds of Native American herbology. In this book you will find some parallels between the spiritual attributes of plants and their medicinal properties. Willow, for example, has long been used both in Indian rituals and medicinally for its cooling and soothing properties. Willow penetrates what is harsh in life and delicately delivers the patient in a ritual setting to a place of peace and equanimity. Today we use salicinin from the willow as the active ingredient in aspirin. It cools the feverish body and delivers us from aches and pains.

Mystics from every tradition know that when a great being dies, his or her fragrance remains for all to share and incorporate. In hunting cultures, the sign of man's limitation was his scent. It traveled ahead of his presence, alerting the animals and determining his success in supplying the necessities of life. Burning a sacred plant renders a solid, material entity into its spiritual form, its essence or fragrance. These plants were beautiful in bloom and were consumed by fire— the cleanser; smoke mysteriously disappeared into the great void, the abode of gods and departed spirits, to whom the breath of smoke was sweet.

> To seek favors from the spirit world we must shed our finite nature.

To seek favors from the spirit world we must shed our finite nature. To do this it is necessary to purify ourselves, to lose our scent and replace it with the fragrance of the plant world. Plants are the ideal mediators between man and the supernatural realm. The act of burning plants containing special medicinal properties serves as a message to the spirit world that these qualities are needed here at this time. When we put a prayer into the smoke with our breath, we act within the belief that the purifying fire and the traveling air will help actualize our spiritual intentions. The smoke is sent with the breath, the gift of life, and this is pleasing to the spirit world.

There are many ways to invoke spirit in the ordinary tasks of daily life. This is done by talking to the spiritual essence that lives within and behind ordinary things and events. At points of passage, on paths and at crossroads, we can make offerings and send them to the Great Spirit with smoke. On the occasion of crossing a threshold, entering and exiting through the doors of our houses or special rooms, these simple acts can bring spirit into a place in time. The creation of a magical portal, the rite of passing through the door, can be easily achieved with an altar affixed to the door and sacred smoke. We say, "May the Great Spirit preserve thy going out and thy coming in from this time forth evermore."

In the morning time, we greet that which moves within and behind Sun with an offering of water and smoke of sweet herbs to change the nature of our days into days aligned with spirit. The simple act of greeting the rising Sun and giving thanks to the setting Sun strengthens our connection to spirit; we invite the mystery of the unseen worlds into our lives.

In times of passage, when departing from a familiar place, when embarking into the unknown, and when entering into new territory, use incense upon entering and exiting your vehicle. Your car is a magical object because it takes you every day from home into the unfamiliar. Times of transition are times of uncertainty. The use of incense with prayers in an automobile sets your spiritual course or intention for the day: when leaving a job or loved one; when leaving one home for another; upon setting out toward first things, new work or new relationships.

Intermediate zones have significance to spirit.

On our daily walks and hikes, upon crossing rivers or mountain passes, crossing intermediate regions bordering field and forest, we can make offerings. Intermediate zones have significance to spirit. In times of inspiration or communion with the spirit of a place, we can give thanks with a bundle of herbs, a special rock, or a stake adorned with a sheaf of straw placed on the path or beside it. This lets other travelers know that this is a holy place where something out of the ordinary has occurred in our hearts or minds. It may take time for us to see things this way, but with practice we add dimension and texture to our daily lives. Before long, we are gifted with a different kind of soul sustenance.

Collectively, we remember certain kinds of rites that our ancestors performed, which, if resurrected in accordance with our own aesthetics and circumstances, add beauty to our lives and bring us closer together.

There is no greater prayer than gratitude.

In old times, strangers were sacred beings, endowed with magical properties, supernaturally benevolent or malevolent. Rites of incorporation of a stranger generally involved the visitor in identifying himself with those he met. In historical times travelers came exhausted and hungry; they were greeted with food, water and a smoke of tobacco. Welcoming the traveler can be consecrated in a simple gesture sent to Spirit with the smoke of sacred plants.

Imagine how our lives would change if we made simple gestures of welcome: to the new child in the classroom; to honor new neighbors or new collaborators or travelers from distant lands; to reestablish connections with old friends after a time of disagreement; to mark times of passage between old partnerships and new ones.

There is no greater prayer than gratitude. Things remain the same until the day we find ourselves grateful for things as they are. We may use ceremonial smoke to invoke protection and magic, but first and foremost we use it to give thanks as in this prayer of the Iroquois:

We return thanks to our mother, the earth,
    which sustains us.
We return thanks to the rivers and streams,
    which supply us with water.
We return thanks to all herbs,
    which furnish medicines
    for the cure of our diseases.
We return thanks to the corn,
    and to her sisters,
    the beans and squashes, which give us life.
We return thanks to the bushes and trees,
    which provide us with fruit.
We return thanks to the wind, which,
    moving the air,
    has banished diseases.
We return thanks to the moon and stars,
    which have given to us their light
    when the sun has gone.
We return thanks to our grandfather He-no,
    that he has protected his grandchildren from
    witches and reptiles,
    and has given to us his rain.
We return thanks to the sun,
    that he has looked upon the earth
    with a beneficent eye.
Lastly, we return thanks to the Great Spirit,
    in whom is embodied all goodness,
    and who directs all things
    for the good of his children.

Part I

The Use of Sacred Plants in Ceremony

The Use of Sacred Plants in Ceremony

The Ancestors Help Us to Practice

In most indigenous cultures there is no word for "art" distinct from the acts of making beauty in the routines of daily life. In contemporary western culture, each of us can perform as "artists" in our most healing capacity by remaking ordinary time and space into extraordinary time and space through simple ritual and ceremony. In the Native American ritual forms outlined below, we see into the spiritual foundations that create the transformative elements of traditional ceremonies. It is important to ground our personally created rituals by studying how the ancestors did this work. As westernized people we have our own kinds of diseases and problems stemming from a sense of separation from the world of plants, animals and spirit. Our alienation from the tribe, our disregard for the knowledge of the ancestors and the well-being of the coming generations, have made us destructive to ourselves and other beings. On the positive side, it has rendered us emotional pioneers, moving toward individuation of distinct personalities and skills. But in this process of pioneering we have become strangely formed, lop-sided creatures. A young western girl or boy has less of a psychic blueprint to follow in order to grow into a noble man or woman representative of their culture. Today, we must learn discernment and wisdom to prioritize our values and choose our behaviors according to the best of what the entire world has to offer. When we study traditional spiritual practices, we do so with an eye toward authentic adaptation, in order to live wisely and beautifully when faced with contemporary challenges.

Recreating ordinary time and space into extraordinary time and space begins with a momentous occasion: birth, puberty, death or a crisis of need. We begin by peering into the universal aspect of the occasion demanding human connection with the Great Spirit. Our intent or motivation becomes the spine of the ceremony. In the words of Tsalagi (Cherokee) medicine woman, Dhyani Ywahoo, there are "rituals for purifying ignorance and obstruction; for clarifying the mind, for pacifying afflicting emotions, illusions and suffering; for magnetizing the good, and for actualizing the vision of peace and harmony held as a sacred ember within the heart of every being." We choose the elements of our rituals: appropriate time, space, power objects, participants, colors and costume, all of which live in symbolic resonance with our intent.

Our personal wounds and crisises have universal aspects.

Our personal wounds and crisises have universal aspects. A ceremony may be designed as the occasion to ask for forgiveness, to make a sacrifice, to purify oneself and make a pact with the Great Spirit to change oneself. Our mistakes are symptomatic of common hindrances to growth: abuses of power, trespasses into someone else's territory, dishonesty, thieving. These mistakes are symptomatic of greed, hatred, and ignorance. Every personal/universal story seeking redemption may be symbolically linked to places where people likewise suffer. Man-made institutions such as laboratories, corporations, prisons, mental hospitals, or old battle grounds are places where several basic universal forms of suffering are personalized in various ways. For our ceremonies, we may choose a quiet, untraveled locale in proximity or within view of these symbolic sites, or we may choose to do our prayers quietly within the workplace or domicile where these abuses commonly occur. For example, a prayer spoken quietly in the restroom at work or in the privacy of our offices, sent to spirit with incense, can set into motion the intent to speak honestly throughout the day in challenging circumstances.

We choose our temenos, the sacred site, as a place that symbolically represents the theme of our objective. When choosing outdoor sites for ceremony we take both practical, spiritual and geomantic considerations into mind. A place needs to be both private, safe and secure. Logistics need to be examined before going too far off the trail; we don't want to get lost or disappear from our support system.

If we have time to observe the Chinese principles of feng shui in choosing an auspicious and powerful spot in nature, we can follow some basic rules of thumb. Sacred space involves recognition of alignment in the cosmos. A compass can help us to fix our coordinates with north, south, west and east. In the forest we can trace a line connecting all the brightest green plants. Such lush stripes are called "dragon veins" or "green ribbons." When we walk through wilderness with our eyes opened we all retain the half-forgotten capacity to recognize special and magical places. All it takes is our intent and we will remember. We may look for shapes on the landscape suggestive of animals or objects. Hills and mountains resembling animals and objects contain powers and characteristics of those animals. Feng shui practices work because they have been a part of our lives for many ages, and our minds are powerful enough to revive these relationships between self and place.

Many mountain ranges appear as dragons with lines of ridges leading to a summit as linking vertebrae. With a map we can choose a site at the proper anatomical part of the dragon. We don't want to set up camp just under his mouth or nostrils, for example. Auspicious spots lie close to veins of subterranean energy delineated by points, "dragon pores" of rich green foliage and vegetation. These dragon veins run down the ridges and backs of mountains, following the nerve network. With our map or our eyes alone we may examine the contours of mountains and the course of streams. We face east and north to meditate, south and east to build our homes. We look for rounded hills and gentle valleys; large old trees; large, oddly shaped stones. Flat, riverless plains are devoid of energy. Meandering rivers are preferable to straightened ones. The most auspicious spot of all for meditating and building is in the lap of a rock or mountain formation that is like a giant armchair, preferably with the protection of a stone or hillock like a footstool before it.

> Sacred time is a symbolic thing that connects all cultures, and all of our ancestors.

Sacred time is a symbolic thing that connects all cultures, and all of our ancestors. Ceremonies are more apt to work if we take time to choose an auspicious time, simply because humans have always done this throughout history. A solar eclipse has different significance than a lunar eclipse, which has a different significance than our birthdays, our death anniversaries, equinoxes, solstices or the time of the first menstrual period. Yearly anniversaries are powerful because of the nature of fruition. We all have experienced how certain events naturally cycle in the annual time frame. For example, we are sometimes surprised by the onset of grief until we remember it is the yearly anniversary of the death of a friend. Or, we see projects and ideas return or come into fuller manifestation in a yearly cycle.

We have described how the circle is important to our rituals because of the cycles of nature and nature's tendency toward wholeness or roundness. The circle represents the relationship between the inner and outer worlds. If properly laid with strong intent, it protects us from apparitions and other distracting influences.

It is also important that a ceremony's beginnings and endings are thoughtfully planned and thoroughly performed. Every element of the ceremony—its design, gathering and assembly of materials, words, need to be worked out with consideration of the spiritual source behind all things.

We highlight the use of incense in the following ceremonies so that we can more fully understand the nature of these plants and the relationship of traditional peoples to these offerings. The limbic system which holds our most primary instinctual natures, our deepest memories and the reptilian brain, are immediately aroused by the sense of smell. So, the burning of sacred plants links our primary memories and our deepest creature selves to the highest spiritual aspects of our humanity. This is one of the reasons why fragrant smoke from medicinal plants is so central and effective in transforming ordinary space and time into extraordinary space and time.

Prayers for First Things

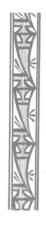

The Birth of Things
Morning Prayers

Morning has broken like the first morning,
Blackbird has spoken like the first bird.
Praise for the singing! Praise for the morning!
Praise for them springing fresh from the Word.

Sweet the rain's new fall sunlit from heaven,
Like the first dew fall on the first grass.
Praise for the sweetness of the wet garden,
Sprung in completeness where His feet pass.

Mine is the sunlight! Mine is the morning!
Born of the one light Eden saw play.
Praise with elation, praise every morning,
God's recreation of the new day!

—Eleanor Farjean

Dhyani Ywahoo, a medicine woman from the Tsalagi (Cherokee) tradition describes ways to use incense to bring blessings to our daily lives. She asks:

> What is praying? To arise in the morning and to thank the sun. To burn sweet grass and sage and cedar, to make tobacco offerings—to acknowledge the beauty of what is, that we may ever be clear in that reflection, that we be firm and not rash, that we be true in our knowing.
>
> And then, at midday, when the sun is overhead, thank all those who have come before and filled your life, filled your body with the energy to be. And, as the sun descends over the western horizon, say, 'Thank you. Oh, a day has passed and another day shall come. I am thankful.'

First Rituals

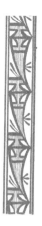

Prayers and Incense Offerings at Birth, Separation from the Mother, Baby-Naming

Pregnancy ceremonies, like those of childbirth, include a great many rites whose purpose is to facilitate delivery and to protect mother and child. ·

Maggie Wilson describes in an article called "Naming Beverly's Baby" the use of juniper in protection of the baby in the nineteen days before the Navajo naming ceremony:

> In a resonant voice that reverberates throughout the village, the dance plazas and passageways of this stone and adobe community, the crier extends an invitation to all the villagers to join the feast honoring the newest member of Shungopavi. While the feast is the culmination of the baby naming ceremony, the rituals actually begin at the time of the baby's birth when two perfect ears of "Mother Corn" are placed on either side of his tiny head. For the next 19 days, the corn stays beside him. While in seclusion he and his mother will

not see direct sunlight and will not be left unattended. During this time both mother and child are considered vulnerable to insidious thought, and, though it is seldom mentioned, the evil acts of malevolent Two-Hearts—people who look and act for the most part like others, but have a dark side. Each day, the baby is bathed and sprinkled with ashes of juniper wood, the common bulwark against adversity, which also serves as a baby powder. "The ashes also prevent rashes and aid the baby's peeling process," says Beverly. On the 19th day, considered to be the most vulnerable of the post-partum period, a line of juniper ashes is streaked onto each of four walls. (In some villages, the ashes are put on the four walls and a ceiling beam on the first day and removed one at a time every fourth day.) Beverly drinks a tea made of juniper branchlets boiled in water and is given a steam bath with the remaining tea. "It helps a mother slim down her insides after giving birth," an aunt explains.

In *Prayers of Smoke*, Barbara Means Adams describes the birth and the making of the sacred umbilical pouch in the Makah tribal tradition:

> At the birth, all the people remain silent and keep their mouths shut, respectful of the baby's niya (one of the four parts of the soul, the breath). All the lights are low. When the contractions are coming quickly, the woman squats and braces herself against a pole. A woman chosen to escort the child into the world holds the baby's head so that the entrance into the world is gentle and

not too fast. She clears the baby's respiratory passages and lays it on the mother's stomach. Then she gently massages the newborn with pure oil. When the baby's navel cord falls off, it goes into the turtle-shaped pouch, along with sweet grass, kinnikinnik, sage and cedar. A boy's pouch is pinned to the shoulder of his shirt. A girl's pouch is pinned to the inside of her dress. The newborn immediately hears lullabies telling of magnificent exploits in hunting and war. Everyone tells the child about the model his or her mother had chosen and about the greatness of that person.

Rites of Initiation, Rites of Passage

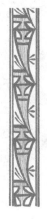

Sweet grass, sage, tobacco and cedar are used by the Oglala Sioux for purification in six of the seven rites:

The Keeping of The Soul

The Inipi Rite of Purification or Sweat Lodge;

Crying for a Vision

Wiwanyag Wachipi or the Sun Dance

Hunkapi, The Making of Relatives Rite

Ishna Ta Awi Cha Lowan, Preparing a Girl For Womanhood Rite.

The term "twice born" clearly indicates the true role of rites of passage. When circumstances or personal choices bring us to the brink of dying to the old ways and being reborn again, we can initiate ourselves with rites of passage symbolically linked to the ancestral ways of doing things.

Traditionally the first initiation rite occurs at times that mark the onset of social or physical puberty. At that time we endure rites of separation from the asexual world, which are usually followed by rites of incorporation into the world of sexuality and, in all societies and all social groups, into a group confined to persons of one sex or another.

Sweet grass, sage and cedar are used by the Makah and the Oglala Sioux, in Coming of Age ceremonies for boys and girls.

Preparing for Womanhood

From the time a Lakota girl child is eight or nine, grandmothers and grandfathers begin the Hunkapi, the preparation for the menstrual cycle. A grandmother is chosen and paid to accompany the child wherever she goes until her marriage. Watching over the girl child, grandmother acts as the Bear, the protector of virgins. A grandfather is chosen and given gifts in honor of his gift of time. He will spend many nights over the course of a year doing vision fasting on behalf of the girl initiate. In these vision fasts he receives instruction as to the child's nature and destiny; information on special diet, her colors, animal helpers and clothing may be received and instructions to prepare her for her role in the tribe.

When the young virgin has her first menstruation period, we make a celebration marking the end of Hunkapi. The girl with her closest family members and the elder man and woman, her protector guides, do a sweat lodge ceremony. At the sweat lodge, grandmother sings a song to invoke the Bear, the protector of virgins. At this sweat lodge

Grandmother sings a song to invoke the Bear, the protector of virgins.

ceremony the elders give the young girl advice received on her behalf in their vision quests. After the sweat lodge there is a feast and ceremony of gift giving from the family to the grandfather and grandmother who have taken the spiritual responsibility of vision fasting for the child.

The next ceremony is the presentation of the feather from the breast of the spotted eagle. It is called "Ishna" and is a preparation for marriage and childbirth. It is a ceremony for the entire community. It begins with the ritual purification of the young woman's new clothing over smoke of sweet grass and sage. She is helped into her new clothing and her face is painted in red symbolizing rebirth. Then four men bring a bear robe and carry the young woman on it. They speak at length about her ancestors, detailed stories about the lives of her family. The young girl is praised by members of the community. The four men burn sage and sweet grass above the young woman's body, and she receives a stalk of corn, a symbol of the making of relatives. This is a ceremony she will perform later in life. The young woman leads the tribe in a circular, clockwise dance. This is a ritual that takes place outdoors, usually in August. She hears for the first time her own honor song, a song just for her that will be sung every time she is honored and remembered, and sung for the last time on the days following her death. At this time she receives the plume from the breast of the spotted eagle. This symbolizes her virginity. On the day she loses her virginity she puts the plume aside for someone else.

Preparing for Manhood

A young Lakota male initiate sacrifices his own eagle, a bird that he has cared for and raised for months before the sacrifice. From this eagle the young male removes all the feathers and puts the head atop a staff in honor of all eagles. The boy keeps the eagle headed staff for the rest of his life. He makes the wing bones into flutes for his Sun Dance ceremony. The wings from the eagle will become his fans to spread the smoke of sage and sweet grass. The tail feathers will become the bustle of his dance costume. If he has a vision, he will make a war bonnet from twenty-eight of the eagle's feathers. Only those who have a vision will be leaders; they will make a headdress.

Crying for a Vision Ceremony

In the hanblecheyapi, Crying for a Vision ceremony, tobacco, sage and sweet grass are traditionally used by the Oglala Sioux:

Traditionally, when we seek a vision, we go to an elder with an offering of tobacco. In this meeting, the seeker talks at length to the elder about his intent and need for a vision. Hopefully the elder will agree to accompany us on our vision quest and hold prayers from a distance and in seclusion. During this four day ordeal, while the fasting initiate cries, laments and prays continuously for his people within his medicine circle, an elder sits in vigilance in a prayer lodge near by. Today, people seeking a vision can find support in individuals or groups who have dedicated their lives to guiding others in this traditional rite. The guides don't interfere with the solitude of the initiate but keep in touch with him or her by leaving daily signs that all is OK. These are left in a cairn of rocks set at a mid-point between the watcher and the initiate.

To begin the Crying for a Vision Rite, the vision seeker finds a willow branch and cuts it to the length of his or her own height. This is the ceremonial pole that will stand in the circle's center. It represents the Great Spirit, and the initiates relationship to the Great Spirit. A string of equal length to the prayer pole is used to draw the circumference of the circle. Then standing in the center of the circle, we face the direction in which the sun rises. A willow stick is then placed at the eastward edge of the circle. Then we turn and face the opposite direction, westward where the sun sets. A willow stick is placed there. Then we draw a line between the two markers, defining an east-west axis. Then turning ninety degrees, the initiate faces northward toward the constellation of the Great Bear and its fixed polestar. Another willow stick is placed at the northern rim. Then we turn around and face the opposite direction, south. Place a willow stick on the southern rim and draw a straight line between the north and south markers.

To the center pole we fasten a tobacco bundle and a spotted eagle feather, a symbol of vision. Then we line the circle with sage. The sage will be the bed. Because the seeker never leaves the circle for four days, the sage will collect the wastes. These will be carried away by the seeker's guardians who will replace the soiled sage with fresh leaves when it is necessary.

The circle is the seeker's protection and so we must never leave it though we are sure to meet with tempters in the form of evil spirits and other apparitions. To these temptations and spirits we make offerings of tobacco. We keep our pipe full for these occasions. The pipe stands in a forked branch at the base of the pole marking east with its mouthpiece toward the one crying for a vision. He sits on the western portal facing east. In times of distress and frightening visitations, the seeker can also make offerings of sweet grass or sage which will defend him. His songs and smoke offerings are powers that make apparitions disappear.

For the duration of the four days and into the nights he sings and prays for his people. He thinks about them continuously and surveys his life and deeds. It is not enough for us to sing for ourselves, we must keep our people always in our heart or mind or the vision quest means nothing to the spirit world. We cry and lament for a vision while fasting. We concentrate on the pole that stands at the center. The seeker must be focused, single-minded and strong.

At the end of the vision quest we must be careful how we reenter the world and use our experience in our daily lives. Skillful reincorporation more fully insures that we will carry out our vision, the spirit world's prescription for changing our life.

The Sweat Lodge Ceremony

We use willow, cedar, sage, sweet grass and tobacco in the Sweat Lodge ceremony.

For the Blackfoot Indians, sweat lodges are associated with all of the ceremonial bundles, with most of the societies, with all of the medicine pipes, and with the Holy Lodge, or Okan, of the Sun Dance.

First we pick a beautiful site, a place of power and solitude, where no one is likely to disturb the ceremony.

We make a sacred circle. A pit is dug at what will be the center of the lodge. This is where the 28 red hot glowing stones the size of softballs will go, seven by seven, at four times during the ceremony when the leader signals to the fire keeper.

We make a grandmother mound with earth from the sacred stone pit. Twelve feet from the pit is this mound and there we bury offerings as symbols of our prayers. Offerings of sage, sweet grass or cedar go in or on top of the grandmother mound.

The amount of willow sticks used for building the sweat lodge varies according to tradition and ceremony. The Horn Society of the Blackfoot Indians use fourteen willows. The Holy Woman's sweat lodge in the Sun Dance is made of one hundred willows, which are gathered by members of the Pigeon Society. Medicine Pipes uses fourteen.

The Oglala Sioux build their sweat lodge of 16 willow sticks, symbolic of transformation. It looks like an inverted basked covered with hides or blankets and tarps, with an eagle feather attached to the crown of the dome.

We sharpen the wands at both ends. One end is planted in the ground, and the wand is woven through the rest of the wands until the other end reaches the ground, where it is forced in.

The Blackfoot and other Plains Indian tribes use *Artemisia ludoviciana* to cover the floor of the sweat lodge and for cleansing. Sage is chewed by the participants during the sweat lodge rituals to relieve thirst because we are not allow to drink water. We wipe the sweat from our bodies with this sage.

Ten paces to the east of the lodge we make the fire for heating the stones till they are red hot and barely discernible as rocks. The fire is made on sticks laid east to west crossed with sticks laid north to south and a tipi of sticks placed over the top of them. The leader says prayers before lighting the fire and makes offerings of sweet grass, cedar, tobacco and sage.

After we build the lodge and the fireplace, with the red hot stone pit and grandmother mound in place, but before the people enter, the leader comes in through the eastern flap and crawls around clockwise to his place to the right of the door. From there he consecrates the space and his pipe by purification prayers and the smoke of burning sweet grass.

He then leaves the lodge and props the pipe against the grandmother mound with the bowl facing west and the stem facing east.

At sundown, the leader enters first. All motion goes clockwise. He crawls all the way around and sits cross-legged by the door.

Then the guest of honor comes in crawling clockwise with his gourd rattles and takes his place on the west side of the lodge facing the door flap.

Then the others crawl in and fill in clockwise. After everyone is seated, four stonepeople, representing the four directions, are brought in and sprinkled with cedar. Then three additional stones, totaling seven red hot fire balls, are brought in to make the first round. Then the flap comes down and everyone is in the womb of Mother Earth, naked and humble as the space fills with heat and the sound of the gourd rattling and the drum beating.

In the first round of prayers, sage, sweet grass and cedar fill the air.

In the first round of prayers, sage, sweet grass and cedar fill the air. The first round of prayers may be dedicated to those who made the sweat lodge possible, or they may be dedicated to the four directions.

Then the leader pours water over the stones. Everyone focuses on the rattles to move easily into a trance. Prayers and songs begin with each person to the left of the leader on the south-southeast side of the door. The prayer stick goes round and each person sings or prays.

All four rounds continue in the same way. You can dedicate each round to themes of each direction beginning with the south, continuing to the west, north and east. Then by the fourth round the tobacco pipe is passed and smoked. After all have smoked, the sweat lodge is over.

The sweat lodge is a place that induces profound purification and vision. We visit with our ancestors. We see animal helpers. Prayer should be dedicated to the good of all beings or the spirit world may not take it seriously.

The Sun Dance

In the Cheyenne Wiwanyag Wachipi, the Sun Dance, we offer our bodies and souls to Wakan-Tanka. This sacred dance marathon, lasting four days and four nights, is accompanied by singing, drumming and offerings accompanied by the smoke of sacred plants. The flesh of the dancer's bodies are attached by thongs to the cottonwood tree that stands in the center. The dancers dance for four days toward and back from the cottonwood tree until the Great Spirit dances through us and for us. In this ecstatic state all of the dancers eventually break free from the thongs, one by one, sacrificing flesh without pain to Wakan-Tanka. In this ceremony, all the old and holy men gather; a large tipi is built and sage is placed all around inside it. Along with a Chanunpa, we bring the following sacred objects:

twist tobacco	a tanned buffalo calf hide
bark of the red willow	rabbit skins
sweet grass	eagle plumes
sage	blue paint
a flint ax	rawhide
buffalo tallow	a buffalo skull
a rawhide bag	whistles from the wing bones
eagle tail feathers	of the spotted eagle

We use tobacco both in preparation for the Sun Dance ceremony and throughout the dance's duration. The priest chooses a cottonwood tree and marks it with sage. Then the scouts pretend to search for themselves in the four directions for the right tree. Upon finding the cottonwood tree that will stand as the center pole for the dancers, the scouts bless it with tobacco and this prayer:

Of all the many standing peoples, you O rustling cottonwood have been chosen in a sacred manner; you are about to go to the center of the people's sacred hoop, and there you will represent the people and will help us to fulfill the will of Wakan-Tanka. You are a kind and good-looking tree; upon you the winged peoples have raised their families; from the tip of your lofty branches down to your roots, the winged and four-legged peoples have made their homes. When you stand at the center of the sacred hoop you will be the people, and you will be as the pipe, stretching from heaven to earth. The weak dancers will lean upon you, and for all the people you will be a support. With the tips of your branches you hold the sacred red and blue days. You will stand where the four sacred paths cross—there you will be the center of the great Powers of the universe. May we two-leggeds always follow your sacred example, for we see that you are always looking upwards into the heavens. Soon, and with all the peoples of the world, you will stand at the center; for all beings and all things you will bring that which is good. Hechetu welo!

The priest then offers his pipe to Heaven and Earth, and then with the stem he touches the tree on the west, north, east, and south sides; after this he lights and smoks the pipe.

Sage is used as a wreath around the heads, wrists and ankles of the sundancers.

The Blackfoot dancers wore sage around their wrists and ankles in their Okan (Holy Lodge) of the Sun Dance, as though they were themselves offerings. The Holy Lodge dancer of the Sun Dance performed upon a carpet of juniper branches. An Okan dancer held the wing of an owl in his left hand and a branch of juniper in the other. In addition to carrying the branch, some dancers wore headpieces of juniper berries; the headpiece had seven berries representing the Bunched Stars, (Pleiades).

Black Elk tells us that in "every Sun Dance we wear wreaths of sage upon our heads, for it is a sign that our minds and hearts are close to Wakan-Tanka and His Powers, for the wreath represents the things of the heavens—the stars and planets, which are very mysterious and Wakan."

"Kablaya then told the dancers how they must paint themselves: the bodies were to be painted red from the waist up; the face, too, must be painted red, for red represents all that is sacred, especially the earth, for we should remember that it is from the earth that our bodies come, and it is to her that they return. A black circle should be painted around the face, for the circle helps us to remember Wakan-Tanka, who, like the circle, has no end. . . Then a black line should be drawn from the forehead to a point between the eyes; and a line should be drawn on each cheek and on the chin, for these four lines represent the Powers of the four directions. Black stripes were painted around the wrists, the elbow, the upper part of the arm, and around the ankles. Black, you see, is the color of ignorance, and thus, these stripes are as the bonds which tie us to the earth. You should also notice that these stripes start from the earth and go up only as far as the breasts, for this is the place where the thongs fasten into the body, and these thongs are as rays of light from Wakan-Tanka. Thus, when we tear ourselves away from the thongs, it is as if the spirit were liberated from our dark bodies." (Joseph Epes Brown, *The Sacred Pipe, Black Elk's Account of the Seven Rites of the Oglala Sioux*, p. 52.)

Rites of Last Things

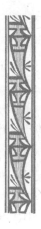

Ceremonies and Prayers for
Keeping of the Soul
and for the Release of the Soul after Death

The Keeping of the Soul Rite

According to Black Elk, as told to Joseph Epes Brown, the Keeping of the Soul Rite is for purifying the soul of the newly dead so that it and the spirit can reunite as one, it can return to the place where it was born and need not wander about the earth as in the case of the souls of bad people. It also brings the hearts of our people more closely together. The occasion of death becomes an occasion through which "our love for one another is increased." Whenever a soul is kept, the people visit the tipi of the departed one and pray together. On the day the soul is released, all the people send their prayers to Wakan-Tanka with the soul who will take these voices with his soul on his sacred path.

The soul that is kept is a messenger to Wakan-Tanka and the touchstone of Wakan-Tanka on earth. The keeper of the soul, often a relative, must speak, see and touch in a sacred manner. He must never fight or use a knife, no matter for what purpose. He must be in prayer at all times and be an example to his people in everything.

Death becomes an occasion through which "our love for one another is increased."

He must raise his head often to look into the heavens. In this way, the relative of the departed becomes a holyman who simultaneously teaches the people and purifies the soul of the departed. Within the tipi where the soul is kept, there is always a woman who has been chosen to care for the sacred bundle. During her sacred duty, she ritually creates sacred food which is kept in a specially painted buffalo-hide box. This is saved for the day when the soul is released. For the duration of soul-keeping, the tribe treats the soul keeper as a holy person, making offerings to him on the occasions of hunting, bringing gifts. The departed holy soul, represented by a lock of hair, purified by sweet grass and wrapped in a hide bundle, lives at the sacred center of the tribe's hoop. In this way the soul becomes the tribe's temple until its release, giving happiness and blessings to whomever comes near it.

Barbara Means Adams describes the use of sage, sweet grass, cedar and tobacco for the Keeping of the Soul ceremony on the occasion of her husband's death:

> The first thing he did was to cut a lock of hair from my husband's forehead. He burned sweet grass to purify the hair. Then he wrapped it in a buckskin bundle and got ready for the public ceremony.
>
> About fifty relatives and friends gathered in our home in Wounded Knee. Everyone sat on the floor in a darkened room. Bill Good Voice Elk burned sage, sweet grass and cedar and passed the soul bundle over the smoke. My husband's drum was hanging on the wall. We all saw

points of light like fireflies dancing over the drum. With each twinkling came a beat. These were Bill Good Voice Elk's helpers. They drummed throughout the ceremony.

My sons and I had prepared tobacco ties, four hundred different-colored ones, as offerings. We presented them. We heard a banging of the screen door, as if a strong wind were battering the house. Bill told us that other souls were coming into the room. It is common for recently departed souls to come back to support someone else who is just entering their realm.

In the talking circle, everyone had a turn verbalizing his or her grief. Everyone asked the purified soul for help in coping with the loss. When the talking was finished, we passed my husband's pipe. The lights came on, and that was the end of the first ceremony.

Black Elk describes the Keeping of the Soul ceremony in the classic book, *The Sacred Pipe*:

A lock of the child's hair was then taken, and as High Hollow Horn did this he prayed:

"O Wakan-Tanka behold us! It is the first time that we do Thy will in this way, as You have taught us through the sacred woman. We will keep the soul of this child so that our Mother the Earth will bear fruit, and so that our children will walk the path of life in a sacred manner."

High Hollow Horn then prepared to purify the child's lock of hair; a glowing coal was brought in, and a pinch of sweet grass was placed upon it.

"O Wakan-Tanka," High Hollow Horn prayed, "this smoke from the sweet grass will rise up to You, and will spread throughout the universe; its fragrance will be known by the winged, the four-leggeds, and the two-leggeds, for we understand that we are all relatives; may all our brothers be tame and not fear us!"

High Hollow Horn took up the lock of hair, and holding it over the smoke, made a motion with it to Heaven, to Earth, and to the four quarters of the universe; then he spoke to the soul within the hair.

"Behold O soul! Where you dwell upon this earth will be a sacred place; this center will cause the people to be as Wakan as you are. Our grandchildren will now walk the path of life with pure hearts, and with firm steps!"

After purifying the lock of hair in the smoke, High Hollow Horn turned to the mother and father of the child, saying: "We shall gain great knowledge from this soul which has here been purified. Be good to it and love it, for it is Wakan. We are now fulfilling the will of Wakan-Tanka, as it was made known to us through the sacred woman; for do you not remember as she was leaving how she turned back the second time? This represents the keeping of the soul, which we are now going to do. May this help us to remember that all the fruits of the winged, the two-leggeds, and the four-leggeds, are really the gifts of Wakan-Tanka. They are all Wakan and should be treated as such!"

The lock of hair was wrapped in sacred buckskin, and this bundle was placed at a special place in the tipi. Then High Hollow Horn took up the pipe, and after holding it over the smoke, filled it carefully in a ritual manner; pointing the stem towards heaven, he prayed.

"Our Grandfather, Wakan-Tanka, You are everything, and yet above everything! You are first. You have always been. This soul that we are keeping will be at the center of the sacred hoop of this nation; through this center our children will have strong hearts, and they will walk the straight red path in a Wakan manner.

"O Wakan-Tanka, You are the truth. The two-legged peoples who put their mouths to this pipe will become the truth itself; there will be in them nothing impure. Help us to walk the sacred path of life without difficulty, with our minds and hearts continually fixed on You!"

The pipe was then lighted and smoked, and was passed sunwise around the circle. The whole world within the pipe was offered up to Wakan-Tanka. When the pipe came back to High Hollow Horn, he rubbed sweet grass over it on the west, north, east, and south sides, in order to purify it lest any unworthy person might have touched it; turning to the people, he then said: "My relatives, this pipe is Wakan. We all know that it cannot lie. No man who has within him any untruth may touch it to his mouth. Further, my relatives, our Father, Wakan-Tanka, has made His will known to us here on earth, and we must always do that which He wishes if we would walk the sacred path. This is the first time that we carry out this sacred rite of keeping the soul, and it will be of great benefit to our children and to their children's children!"

Releasing of the Soul Rite

The family and the soul keeper usually prepare the soul for a year before the Releasing of the Soul Rite. For this ritual, many things have to be gathered by the family of the departed one, so for poor families this may take many years.

The sacred pipe ceremony is most elaborate in this ritual. A sacred tipi is made with a fire at the center, the representative of Wakan-Tanka on Earth.

In the words of Black Elk:

The helper of the keeper of the soul then takes a pipe and holding it up to the heavens he cries:

"This day is Wakan because a soul is to be released. All over the universe there will be happiness and rejoicing! O You sacred Power of the place where the sun goes down, it is a great thing we are doing in placing You in the pipe. Give to us for our rites one of the two sacred red and blue days which You control!"

This Power of the west, now in the tobacco, is placed in the pipe, and holding another pinch of kinnikinnik towards the north, the helper prays.

"O You, Thunderbeing, there where Waziah has his lodge, who comes with the purifying winds, and who guards the health of the people; O Baldheaded Eagle of the north, Your wings never tire! There is a place for You too in this pipe, which will be offered to Wakan-Tanka. Help us, and give to us one of Your two sacred days!"

Then holding another pinch of kinnikinnik to the east, the helper begins to pray.

"O You sacred Being of the place where the sun comes up, who controls knowledge! Yours is the path of the rising sun which brings light into the world. Your name is Huntka, for You have wisdom and are long-winged. There is a place for You in the pipe; help us in sending our voice to Wakan-Tanka! Give to us Your sacred days!"

This Power of the east is placed in the pipe, and then another pinch of kinnikinnik is held towards the south, with the prayer:

"O You who guard that path leading to the place towards which we always face, and upon which our generations walk, we are placing You in this sacred pipe! You control our life, and the lives of all the peoples of the universe. Everything that moves and all that is will send a voice to Wakan-Tanka. We have a place for You in the pipe; help us in sending our vice, and give to us one of Your good days! This we ask of You, O White Swan, there where we always face!"

The stem of the pipe and a pinch of kinnikinnik are then held towards the earth.

"O You, sacred Earth, from whence we have come, You are humble, nourishing all things; we know that You are Wakan and that with You we are all as relatives. Grandmother and Mother Earth who bear fruit, for You there is a place in this pipe. O Mother, may Your people walk the path of life, facing the strong winds! May we walk firmly upon You! May our steps not falter. We and all who move upon You are sending our voices to Wakan-Tanka! Help us! All together as one we cry: help us!"

When the pipe has thus been filled with all the Powers and with all that there is in the universe, it is given to the keeper of the soul, who takes it and, crying as he walks, goes to the tipi of the keeper of the most sacred pipe, to ask him to lead the rites of the releasing of the soul.

Then the keeper of the most sacred pipe makes another elaborate pipe offering of this kind, placing the whole universe inside the pipe, and then, turning to the people, the keeper of the pipe says: "Since we have done all this correctly, the soul should have a good journey, and it will help our people to increase and to walk the sacred path in a manner pleasing to Wakan-Tanka."

Before the soul is released, its spiritual influence or seed is passed along to four virgin girls. First the soul is fed purified, spirit food to sanctify the food and fortify the spirit on his journey. This sanctified holy food becomes spiritually contagious and powerful. As the soul is fed the pipe keeper says, "You are about to eat this Wakan food. When it is placed in your mouth its influence will spread, and it will cause the fruits of our Mother, the Earth, to increase and prosper. Your grandmother is Wakan; upon Her we stand as we place this food in your mouth. Do not forget us when you go forth to Wakan-Tanka! But look back upon us!" The holy food consisting of buffalo meat and cherry juice is purified again with sweet grass and fed to the four virgins so that their fruits and their children will always be Wakan!

Ceremonies and Prayers, the Use of Cedar and Juniper, Before Bedtime

In Dhyani Ywahoo's book: *Voices of our Ancestors*, she passes on the method of dream attentiveness as taught by Grandfather Eona Fisher:

1. Upon retiring to the sleeping chamber, smoke the area with the offering of burning cedar or juniper to the north, east, south, and west and to heaven and earth. The atmosphere around you is composed of thought. When your thought is clarified through mindfulness practice and you take time to smudge the area, to make smoke offerings, you are also giving thanks to Earth for fresh breath and helping to clarify individual and planetary thought.

2. Make a prayer acknowledging yourself as a vehicle of light, giving thanks for the good that has come that day and an affirmation of intent to live in harmony with all your relations.

3. Lie upon your bed and review your actions of the day. In your mind's eye make corrections if necessary. For example, if you neglected to respond from the heart with another person, see yourself relating heart to heart; if you spoke with anger, see yourself speaking compassionately.

4. Count slowly backward from ten to one, affirming that you will remember all that occurs during sleep.

5. Give yourself the task of raising your hands to the sky in the dream, to call forth fruitful life.

6. On awakening, stretch and give thanks, and make note of your dreams in the dream journal.

The Four Directions

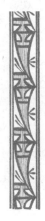

All living things strive toward wholeness. That is why the circle is the most powerful symbol in all Indian cosmologies. Black Elk said, "There is much power in the circle; the birds know this for they fly in a circle, and build their homes in the form of a circle; this the coyotes know also, for they live in round holes in the ground." We believe in eternal recurrence, which is what the circle tells us.

Among many Indian people, a child's first teaching is of the four great powers of the medicine wheel. For the child to grow into an actualized being, living in harmony with other beings, she must become thoroughly familiar with the qualities of each direction. With her heart and mind she must remember to continually touch these qualities, and by touching, to summon their powers throughout her days.

All living things strive toward wholeness.

All beings including the trees, flowers, two and four leggeds grow by filling out toward every way, encompassing and in touch with all directions and, according to the fortune or circumstance of our birth and growth, we become more or less whole. The newborn child is oriented to perceive from a certain perspective.

The southern orientation is the place of innocence and trust, and for perceiving closely our nature of heart. One who perceives from the south knows things of the heart. By touching they feel experience from close proximity. Yellow is the color of the south and the Sun is strongest when facing in that direction. The south continues to deliver to us the gifts of innocence, trust and boundless renewal energy until the day we die, if we honor these qualities. The sacred plants we find on the south of the wheel that can be used for prayers of this orientation are cedar and copal. As we will see in the following pages, cedar is for protection, for new life and is a friend of the Sun. Copal is used for ceremonies with a southwesterly emphasis. According to Tsalagi (Cherokee) medicine woman Dhyani Ywahoo, the south-southwest direction represents the gathering of experience and recognition of responsibility to self and all living creatures; returning sustenance and abundance to others. The southwest represents the spread of family, clan, based on right relationship. The west-southwest is the place where we accept our power and decide to share and carry forth in harmony with the present, giving birth to children of tomorrow, fed by traditions of our grandmothers.

Sacred clowns destroy old forms, institutions, and expectations.

From the west, one perceives through introspection, one learns the shadowy creatures, facets and coursing of one's own mind and psyche, and can turn and transmute these things with one's will. According to Lame Deer, "Everything in nature moves in a certain way that the whites call clockwise. Only the Thunderbeings of the west move in a contrary manner, counterclockwise." Westerly beings are sacred clowns, they destroy old forms, institutions, expectations, they wear their clothing upside down. Black is the color of the west. The sacred plants that consecrate the west and rituals with a western emphasis are mugwort, willow and sage. Some traditions would say that sage is best used in a ceremony that has an eastern emphasis. As a purifier and disperser of unwanted energies, sage does well in ceremonies oriented to themes and qualities of the west. In its western orientation, mugwort is a visionary plant used for clear dreaming and prophesy. It gives strength to astral travelers. In some traditions willow is a totem of the underworld and unconscious.

One receives wisdom by remembering to seek the spiritual root behind all forms.

A person who perceives from the north is a wise person who has learned the hard way. The austere old man from the north has lived through famine, drought, icy snows, plague, flooding, poisoning, wars, loss of family, other kinds of heartbreak, equipment failure, alienation, violation, persecution by strangers. He has led mass migrations through terrible arctic winters, unfamiliar cities, jungle thickets, subterranean haunts. He never wants to make the same mistakes twice. So, he has become a survival master, able to prevent mishap and prepare for adversity through calculation, measuring, objective reasoning. And since these lessons taught him well (he has learned selflessness and the interdependence of all creatures), he deals these lessons from the north. The land is purified of the weak each winter. The plant most sacred to the north is sweet grass. Sweet grass is also called grandmother's hair. Her long white hair is a symbol of experience over time.

The eastern orientation is one of spiritual insight into the origins and causes of things. It has gold star-like clarity that shines and pierces outward. One receives wisdom by remembering to seek the spiritual root behind all forms, problems and circumstances. Plants sacred to the east are the purifying, calming and renewing plants. Pine, and some would assert that sage and tobacco also, belongs to the east of the wheel. Tobacco honors and invokes the departed ancestors; their wisdom comes disembodied from the east. Pine offers peace of mind, fertility and cleansing. It is said that the pine never sleeps, being evergreen, so it is a good watcher over the home.

Each human being combines various ways of seeing and understanding, but to have wisdom without touching, or to have introspection without innocence, or to have innocence without wisdom, is lop-sided. Making offerings of smoke to the directions within a medicine wheel is a way of summoning our innate, hidden attributes. In the formless times, we expressed ourselves as Gods or Living Powers. We had command of all attributes. In the formless times, we lived as pure mind, but this wasn't enough. We chose limitation, incarnation, in order to learn things of the heart through touching. Now it is our work to become whole within the limits of the physical world.

Before beginning any of our other ceremonies, we smudge the people who are going to be present. Smudging is a process of using smoke to clear away any negative energies and to attract positive energies. We use a stone bowl as the container for the sage and sweet grass that we burn. You can smudge with sage, sweet grass, cedar or tobacco. You light the herb with either a coal or a match and blow out the flames so it is smoldering, rather than burning. To keep it smoldering you may fan it with your hand, a feather or a fan.

The person who is doing the smudging first brings the smoke toward his heart and then up over his head. This will help his energy to run in a good direction, and it will take any negative thoughts or feelings from him. He then offers the bowl to the four directions, the Father Sun and the Earth Mother. He takes the bowl around to the people participating. They should be standing in a circle, and the bowl should be taken in a sunwise direction, beginning with the north.

Different peoples begin with different directions. Black Elk begins his prayers from the south and continues west, north, east, returning back to the southern position. He explains:

> Is not the south the source of life, and does not the flowering stick truly come from there? And does not man advance from there toward the setting sun of his life in the west? Then does he not approach the colder north where the white hairs are? And does he not then arrive, if he lives, at the source of light and understanding, which is the east? Then does he not return to where he began, to his second childhood, there to give back his life to all life, and his flesh to the earth whence it came? The more you think about this, the more meaning you will see in it.

A Winnebago Prayer

Hearken, O Earthmaker, our father,
    I am about to offer tobacco to you.
My ancestor concentrated his mind upon you,
    and that with which you blessed him.
    I now ask of you directly.
    I ask for the small amount of life you granted him,
    and for four times the blessings
    you bestowed upon him.
May I never meet with trouble in life.
O Grandfather, chief of the Thunderbirds,
    you who live in the west,
    here is a handful of tobacco.
    Extend to me the deer
    with which you blessed my ancestor.
    I pray to accept this tobacco from me.
May I never meet with trouble in life.
O Grandfathers, northern spirits of the night,
    walkers in darkness,
    to you I offer tobacco
    and ask for the fire places
    which my ancestor received.
    If you smoke this tobacco
    see to it that I never become a weakling.

To you who live in the south,

    you who look like a man,

    you who are invulnerable,

    you who deal out life from one side of your body

    and death from the other,

    you whom we call Disease Giver,

    to you I offer tobacco.

    In daylight, in broad daylight,

    did you bless my ancestor.

    With food you blessed him;

    you told him that he would never fail in anything,

    you told him that you would avoid his home;

    you placed animals in front of him

    that he should have no trouble obtaining them.

An offering of tobacco I make to you

    that you may smoke it

    and that I may not be troubled in life.

From Paul Radin, *Crashing Thunder, The Autobiography of An American Indian*. New York: D. Appleton Co., 1926.

Part II

The Plants of Power

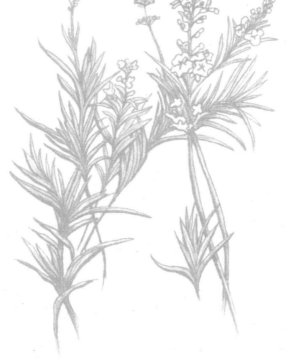

INCENSE CEDAR

Libocedrus decurrens

Incense cedar grows to a vertical height of 50 to 80 feet. It will normally grow at an elevation of about 6000 feet. It has outward spreading branches that may reach an expanse of 96 feet in trees that are over 100 years old.

In Cabalistic lore, cedar is associated with the sephira of Chesed. Chesed is known as Mercy. It is ruled by the planet Jupiter and is associated with the Greek God Zeus.

The genus *Cedrus* has long been considered to be a "God Tree" from the Latin, "deodar." The far-famed Cedars of Lebanon, in the language of prophecy, are frequently employed in the Scriptures as beings of power, prosperity and longevity. The cedar forests are in the mountains of Afghanistan, north Baluchistan and the northwest Himalayas. They also grow in the higher mountains from Nepal up to Kashmir. Over the years the *Cedrus deodar* receives many offerings and homage by wayfarers.

The North American *Cedrus juniperus* can be visited with the same respect. It has been said that their presence will reveal itself and bestow blessings on the traveler. The cedar is often found growing around dry rocky ridges. It may be found from the eastern foothill region of the Rocky Mountains, from Alberta to western Texas, and westward to the coast of British Columbia. It grows from Washington to eastern Oregon, Nevada, and northern Arizona.

The divine nature of the North American cedar conifers has long been understood by the Native Peoples. Cedar is burned while praying either aloud, or silently. Some incense smokes are for attracting good spirits, eliminating negative energie or invoking ancestors. Cedar smoke has been used to create a bridge between heaven and earth and for speaking with the Creator. The power of cedar is well depicted in the Semitic writings of Old World ancestors:

> And so they two came to the cedar forest and stood gazing at its height, looking at the entrance to it where Humbab, the forest guardian, wanders about setting his footsteps. The roads were straight and the way good. The cedars held high there luxurious beauty on the face of the mountain, good was its shade full of pleasure.

In the Sumerian legend of Gilgamesh, the cedar mountain was the abode of gods and the sanctuary of the goddess Irnini. The gods and goddess of this region were Adad, Shamash and Astarte. The Sumerian goddess Astarte was called the "true sovereign of the world," tirelessly creating and destroying, eliminating the old and generating the new. She was worshiped by King Solomon. Cedar was the "tree being" whose attributes matched those of Astarte.

In Egyptian mythology, the cedar is the celestial or cosmic tree. Osiris, as the god of heaven, is frequently identified with cedar, and

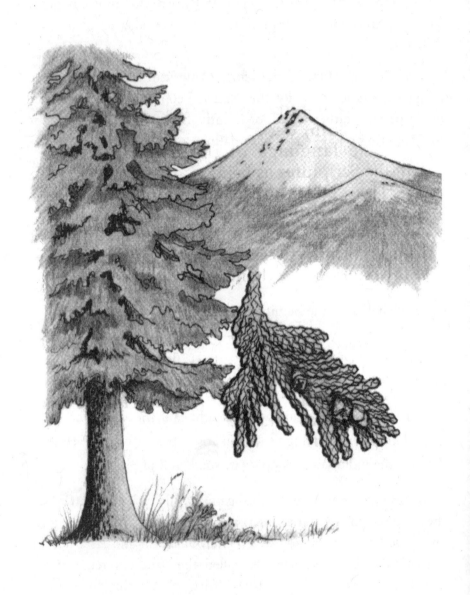

Cedar is the celestial or cosmic tree.

is called the heavenly tree. As ruler of the sky, he can sit in the celestial tree, and can spiritually become one with it. The savior god Osiris is a multifaceted deity, amongst his 200 divine names, he was called Lord of Lords, King of Kings, and God of Gods. He was the Resurrection and the Life, the Good Shepherd, Eternity and Everlastingness. When Osiris grows forth from the cedar tree, he displays his solar nature.

In one version of the Osiris/Isis myth, Isis obtained the coveted cedar column and cut the body of Osiris out of the stem of the tree. The cedar column itself was wrapped in linen, like a mummy, and sprinkled with myrrh. It remained an object of worship at Byblos for nearly three centuries.

Another text describes the initiation of a seer. At one point the initiate descends to the lower world, in meditation. There he sees altars in the waters, tablets of the Gods and the divine cedar tree that is beloved to the Gods.

An ancient Babylonian magical text describes how a man possessed with seven evil spirits can be rid of them. First, he must go to a cedar tree, which shatters the power of the incubus. Then, with the help of an amulet placed on the sick man's head, he must invoke the aid of the Fire God to dispel the seven evil demons.

In North America, cedar is a favorite firewood to the Zuni people, but its most important place is in ceremony. The fibrous bark is shredded and used as tinder to ignite the fire sticks that are made for the New Year fire. At other times firebrands are made of the bark and carried by impersonators of certain gods. The most

Cedar's most important place is in ceremony.

conspicuous gods being "Shu'laawitisi" (Cedar) deputy to the Sun Father.

Cedar is considered an herb of the sun, its element is Fire. It is especially effective for burning at Yule and during winter rituals.

As an incense, cedar purifies an area and banishes nightmares. Native American peoples sometimes burn cedar in sweat lodges to help release heavy emotional energies. Cedar incense is also effective at child blessings and naming ceremonies.

Cedar is burned in sweat lodges to release heavy emotional energies.

Medicinal uses: Aromatic, astringent, diuretic. The twigs may produce abortion, like those of savin, by a reflex action on the uterus. Both fenchone and thujone stimulates the heart muscle. The decoction has been used in intermittent fevers, rheumatism, dropsy, coughs, scurvy, and as an emmenagogue. The leaves, made into an ointment with fat, are a helpful local application in rheumatism. An injection of the tincture into venereal warts is said to cause them to disappear. For violent pains the Canadians have used the cones, powdered, with four-fifths of polypody, made into a poultice with lukewarm water or milk. This is applied to the body, with a cloth over the skin, to prevent any scorching.

Prayer To The Young Cedar   (Kwakiutl)

The woman goes into the woods to look for young cedar trees. As soon as she finds them, she picks out one that has no twists in the bark, and whose bark is not thick. She takes her hand adze and stands under the young cedar tree, and looking upward to it, she prays saying:

> Look at me, friend!
> I come to ask for your dress,
> For you have come to take pity on us;
> For there is nothing for which you cannot be used,
> For you are really willing to give us your dress,
> I come to beg you for this,
> Long-Life maker,
> For I am going to make a basket for lily roots out of you.
> I pray you, friend, not to feel angry
> On account of what I am going to do to you;
> And I beg you, friend, to tell our friends about
>   what I ask of you.
> Take care, friend!
> Keep sickness away from me,
> So that I may not be killed by sickness or in war,
> O friend!

This is the prayer that is used by those who peel cedar bark of young cedar trees and of old cedar trees.

From Franz Boas, *The Ethnology of the Kwakiutl*, p. 130.

RED CEDAR

Juniperus scopulorum

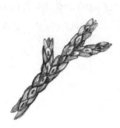

One of nature's most handsome creations, *Juniperus scopulorum*, grows to a great height and spreads its branches horizontally for a considerable distance. The evergreen leaves appear in small tufts like those of the larch.

Red cedar grows between 30 and 40 feet high, with a short, stout trunk sometimes 3 feet in diameter. It often grows divided near the ground into a number of spreading stems. The thick spreading and ascending branches covered with scaly bark. These branches form an irregular round-topped head, and slender four-angled branchlets. At the end of three or four years, they become clothed with smooth pale bark separating later into thin scales. The bark is dark reddish brown or sometimes gray tinged with red. Then the bark is divided by shallow fissures that form into narrow flat connected ridges broken on the surface into persistent shredded scales.

The cedar trees grow on dry rocky ridges. They are also found growing near the coast, usually at elevations of more than 5000 feet. They cover an area from the eastern foothill region of the Rocky Mountains, from Alberta to western Texas, and westward to the coast of British Columbia and Washington. You can also find them growing to eastern Oregon, Nevada and northern Arizona.

Recently-dried, leafy young twigs, contains the bitter principle, pinipicrin, along with tannic acid. They also contain volatile oil,

Prayers rise on cedar smoke and are carried to the Creator.

sugar, gelatinous matter, resin, and thujin. Thujin is a citron-yellow, crystallizable coloring principle, soluble in alcohol. It has an astringent taste and is flammable. It can be split up into glucose, thujigenin and thujetin.

Medicinal uses (like incense cedar): Aromatic, astringent, diuretic. The twigs may produce abortion, like those of savin, by reflex action on the uterus from severe gastrointestinal irritation. Both fenchone and thujone stimulate the heart muscle. The decoction has been used in intermittent fevers, rheumatism, dropsy, coughs, scurvy, and as an emmenagogue. The leaves, made into an ointment with fat, are a helpful local salve for rheumatism. An injection of the tincture into venereal warts is said to cause them to disappear. For violent pain, the Canadians have used the cones, powdered, with four-fifths of polypody. After it is made into a poultice with lukewarm water or milk, it is applied to the body, with a cloth over the skin to prevent any scorching.

In northern America, cedar is burned while praying. The prayers rise on the cedar smoke and are carried to the Creator. Cedar is also spread, along with sage, on the floor of the sweat lodges of some tribes. Many Northwest Indians brush the air with cedar branches to cleanse a home during the House Blessing ceremony. In the Pacific Northwest, the people burn cedar for purification in much the same way as sage. It drives out negative energy, and brings in good influences. The spirit of cedar is considered very ancient and wise, by Pacific Northwest tribes. Old, downed cedar trees are always honored with offerings and prayers.

COPAL

Bureseru microphylla

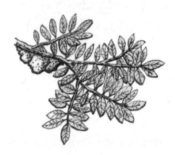

Copal is pitch from trees that are sacred to the Maya Indians. It is likely that copal was gathered often from trees struck by lightning. These places would then become sacred after the visitation by Thunderbeings.

The *Popul Vuh* is a book considered by the Mayan peoples to be a "seeing instrument." It is one of the four sacred books that survived the Auto da Fé book burning, led by missionaries at the time of the Spanish Inquisition. In the *Popul Vuh*, the rhythms of time are described. Mayan deities and their works are illuminated in the book. The incense copal figures prominently in the text, as an offering worthy of attention from the Gods.

Copal was considered a substance very sacred to the Maya. Even to this day at the wayside shrines of Momostenango, Chichicastenango, and the holy mountain of Patohil, the incense is never touched by the human hand once it sits upon the altar. A wooden stick is used to stir the burning copal or to move stray pieces of it into the fire.

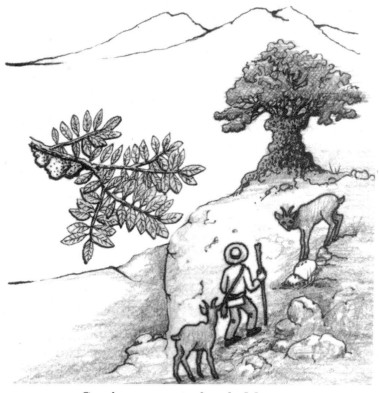

Copal trees are sacred to the Maya.

Copal is always burned during divination and gives nourishment to the gods at the household altars and throughout initiation ceremonies. The daykeeper diviner will cast lots of coral seeds and crystals along a picture of the days of the 260 day calendar. This is to forecast a sequence of events for the future. As copal burns, the daykeeper chants:

> Just let it be found, just let it be discovered, say it, our
> ear is listening, may you talk, may you speak, just find
> the wood for the carving and sculpting by the builder,
> sculptor. Is this to be the provider, the nurturer when

it comes to the planting, the dawning? You corn ker-
nels, you coral seeds, you days, you lots, may you suc-
ceed, may you be accurate.

Copal carries the message to the gods. The Mayan people have
love and reverence for the copal essence, which can be acknowl-
edged in the following myth of origins:

And Jaguar Quittze, Jaguar Night, Mahucutah, and
True Jaguar were overjoyed when they saw the daybring.
It came up first. It looked brilliant when it came up,
since it was ahead of the sun.

After that they unwrapped their copal incense, which
came from the East, and there was triumph in their
hearts when they unwrapped it.

They gave their heartfelt thanks with three kinds at
once:

"Mixtam Copal is the name of the copal brought by
Jaguar Quitze."

"Cauiztan Copal is the name of the copal brought by
Jaguar Night."

"Godly Copal, as the next one is called, is brought by
Mahucutah."

The three of them had their Copal, and this is what
they burned as they incensed the direction of the rising
sun. They were crying sweetly as they shook their burning Copal, the precious Copal.

Copal grows from the Sonora Desert to southern Mexico in dry arid regions. The Burseraceae is a large plant family that extends throughout various climates and ecozones, often with aromatic resins. The black and gold copals are natural pitch resin extrusions gathered by farmers and herders in their off season. The white copal is harvested in the springtime by making scarification marks on the tree. Resin comes from these marks, is collected, heated and poured onto a banana leaf to make a flat loaf shape.

It is known that the Mayan and Aztec dentists filled the teeth of the royal families with copal, to invest their speech with divine clarity. Copal is still used today in dentistry to keep the silver amalgam from discoloring. In Hispanic communities of North America, copal is burned in the Dia de Los Muertos, (Day of the Dead), November 1-4, as a food for the departed relatives. The food helps to sustain them, as they journey into the spirit realm.

Modern investigators have observed that copal has properties that positively influence the immune response of the human body. The immune system preserves the integrity of an individual, protecting one from external, decadent elements.

Travelers Prayer with An Offering of Copal

O God, O lord of the mountains and valleys,
    I have offered you a bit of your food, your drink.
And now I continue on,
    beneath your feet and your hands, I, a traveler.
It cannot hurt you, it cannot grieve you
    to give me plenty of game, big game, small game,
O my father. For you have much.
You have trogons, pheasants, boars.
Show them, reveal them.
Take them and set them in my path.
I will see them and find them,
    for I am beneath your feet,
    beneath your hands: I am fortunate,
    O lord of the mountains,
    O lord of the valleys.
    By your will, your name, and your being,
    all things are abundant.
May I share in them all.
Today, perhaps, I must eat my tortillas,
    and yet I am in rich hunting lands.
    I hope God can see that there are
    no living creatures about.
    Perhaps I will get,
    perhaps I will catch just one little trogon.
    I will see it, I will find it,
    O God, O Mother, O Father.
This is my word and my thought.

Though what I have brought along
for you to eat, for you to drink,
is neither good nor much,
nevertheless my words, my
thoughts, are these, O Mother, O Father.
Now I will sleep beneath your feet,
beneath your hands,
O lord of the mountains and valleys,
O lord of the trees, O lord of the creeping vines.
Again tomorrow there will be day,
again tomorrow there will be light.
I know not where I will be.
Who is my mother? Who is my father?
Only you, O God.
You watch me, guard me, on every path,
through every darkness, and before each obstacle
that you might hide or take away,
O God, my lord,
O lord of the mountains and valleys.
My words, my thoughts, are these. I may have said
too much, or not enough.
You will endure, you will forgive my error.

Kekchi Maya

JUNIPER

Juniperous ssp.

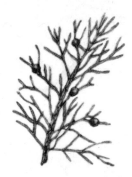

The Juniper is a small shrub, 4 to 6 feet high, and it is widely distributed throughout the Northern Hemisphere. It occurs freely on the slopes of chalk downs and on healthy, siliceous soils where a little lime occurs. It is a common shrub found growing in bands of limestone.

The principal constituent of juniper is the volatile oil, with resin, sugar, gum, water, lignin, wax and salines. The oil is most abundant just before the perfect ripeness and darkening of the fruit.

In many cultures, juniper has been utilized to create an environment that is safe and oftentimes more sacred. The aromatic properties of juniper are used to fight against bad magic, plague and various negative influences. In Greek cosmology, the spirit of the goddess-physician, Artemis, inhabits the juniper. The tenth century ancestors of the Lithuanian people include stories of juniper in their forest mythology. In Pueblo cultures, the leaves are carried in pouches and on our clothes. They are often the only protection or medicine, carried by the Tewa Indians. Today, in the northern

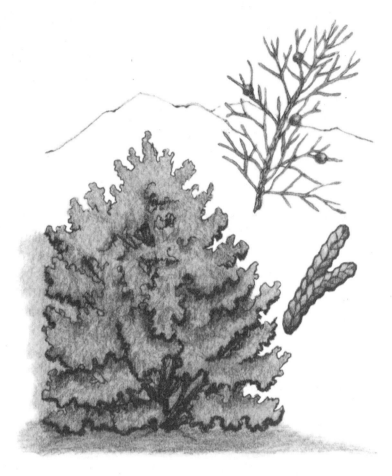

Juniper creates an environment that is safe and sacred.

provinces of China, the burning berries of the juniper purify the air in sick rooms, and prevent the spread of infection.

In ceremonials, the plant serves to dispel negative forces from the environment. In its medical uses, the volatile oil expels toxins from the body and tones the eliminating systems. For these reasons the incense of juniper may be considered a banishing smoke. The nature of the plant may be understood as a purgative.

Juniper knots burn slowly, and will give off a clear smoke, which is why it is desired for feasting and ceremonial fires and is frequently used in fires. When a patient was celebrating the recovery of a long illness, the medicine man and his assistants will make gestures of "throwing the disease away."

Navajo women put a bracelet of dried juniper berries on the babies before they put them to bed. These beads are called "ghost beads," and they keep their children from having bad dreams. To make the ghost beads, the mothers scatter the fresh ripe berries over tall anthills. After several minutes, the busy ants will eat out the center, leaving the desired perforation necessary for stringing the beads.

In the Navajo ceremonials, "Gad bika'igii" is used as an emetic. The juniper is ingested, and the initiate is purified by vomiting. Juniper is also used for making many ceremonial items.

The Arapaho call juniper "the prickly one" or "Bat-they-naw." To cure smallpox, the juniper needles were ground for a scent and thrown on a hot stove or hot rocks, for an infusion.

The Shoshone call the juniper "Sammabe," the "Washo Paal." Medicine people from these tribes, as well as the Paiute, used juniper branches and leaves to cure rheumatism. First they burned the fire down to coals, then they put green juniper boughs on the coals. Then they ask the patient to lie down on the boughs and steam. Meanwhile, the patient drinks a tea made from juniper leaves.

Animals agree about the medicinal properties of juniper.

The Navajo use juniper for a variety of medicinal purposes. It is used as a diuretic and emetic as well as medicine for headaches, influenza, stomach aches, nausea, acne, spider bites and postpartum pain.

In France, the berries of juniper are used as a remedy for chest complaints and in leucorrhoea, blenorrhoea and scrofula.

Animals agree about the medicinal properties of juniper. The fruit is readily eaten by most animals. It helps to prevent and to cure dropsy. When the oil is mixed with lard it makes an excellent salve for exposed wounds and irritation.

The Native Americans will use the leaves either dry, moistened or fresh. They also use the leaves for throwing on hot rocks in saunas and sweat lodges.

Juniper has been a friend to all peoples, in times of famine and drought. The ancestors dried the fruits and stored them for use in wintertime. These berries would later be ground into a meal and used to make mush or cakes. They were sometimes roasted and ground to make a substitute for coffee. Another use they found for the plant was to burn the green leaves, put boiling water on the ashes, and use the strained liquid as a flavoring in various other foods. In times of acute food shortage, the ancestors would sometimes peel off the inner bark of the trunk and chew it to avoid starvation.

There is a tree, in Logan Canyon, Utah, called the Jardine Juniper. It is estimated to be fifteen hundred years old. To gather power and secure a relationship with the spirit of the plant, you can visit this tree and speak its many names:

Ooss moapa P.! Sammabe Sho! Poosh! Tsekie sino kosa!
And its Old world names: *Ginepro! Enebro! Genevrier!*

LAVENDER

Lavandula officianalis

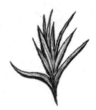

Lavender, known by its folk names Elf Leaf, Nard, Nardus and Spike, is botanical Lavandual, a genus of the natural order Labiatae (lip like petals). It is distinguished by an egg-shaped tubular calyx. Lavender has four stamen that bend downward.

The genus of Lavender includes about three dozen species, all native to the Mediterranean countries and India. This bushy evergreen under shrub is two feet high, with spiking whorls of beautiful blush violet flowers. It has an affinity for crystalline rocks, barren soils, and coastal areas elevated above the fog level. It survives in intense summer heat and bitter cold, where few plants can survive.

The alchemists believed that lavender was ruled by Mercury, a neutral, androgynous planet being. They, and the homeopathic physicians, saw lavender's mediating or conciliatory effect helping to balance extreme conditions. It balances toxicity and crisis of mental derivation with a liberating and calming influence. Lavender's graceful survival within adversity is a reflection of its mercurial or transforming, fire-like properties. The volatile oil of

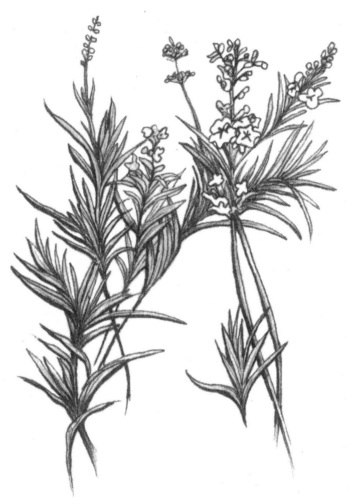

Lavender restores balance, whether of mind or body.

lavender belongs to the fire element group, and so it is known to express Mercury's properties through the sign of Leo. Lavender soothes and calms the nerves and stimulates the healing process.

The healing spirit of Mercurius moves between the opposite polarities of poison and panacea, strain and mercy, crisis and grace. The fragrance of lavender imparts a feeling of inner freedom that allows one to let go of compulsions, anger and other bad habits of mind. *Salmon's Herbal* says:

It is good also against the biting of serpents, mad-dogs and other venomous creatures, being given inwardly and applied poultice-sie to the parts wounded. The spirituous tincture of the dried leaves or seeds, if prudently given, cures hysteric fits though vehement and of long standing.

It was formerly believed that the asp, a dangerous kind of viper, made the lovely lavender its habitual abode. The plant had to be constantly approached with great caution.

Throughout the ages, lavender is used in love spells and in sachets. Clothing rubbed with the fragrance of flowers will attract love. Our great-great grandmothers may have rubbed the purplish blue petals on their paper when writing love notes. The scent of lavender particularly attracts men. Lavender water or the essential oil was worn by many prostitutes, to both advertise their profession, as well as attract new customers. North African women use lavender to guard against any maltreatment, especially from their husbands.

The nature of lavender's conciliatory work sheds light on its dual traditional uses. It promotes love, and guards chastity. It frees the subject from too much contemplation about a loved one. Lavender has long been associated with spiritual love. The medieval abbess, composer and physician, Hildegarde Von Bingen recommended lavender for maintaining a pure character.

Sometimes, the flowers of lavender are burned or smoldered to induce sleep and rest, and can be scattered about the home to maintain a feeling of peacefulness. The plant is so powerful that if one becomes depressed and gazes upon it, all sorrow will depart and a joyous feeling will override the depression. Indeed, the odor of lavender was thought to be beneficial for longevity.

Wild lavender's healing power is extremely diverse, partly due to its complex combination of chemical substances. About 160 different substances in the plant have been identified, but chemists are certain that many more exist. Its versatile effects range from analgesic through antidepressant, antiseptic, bactericidal and vermifuge. Its properties can be described as calming, soothing, and most importantly, balancing.

This ability to restore balance, whether of mind or body, is lavender's most important quality. The restored balance generates an atmosphere conducive for healing. In the *British Pharmacopoeia of 1860*, it was said to be useful, "against the falling sickness, and all cold distempers of the head, womb, stomach, and nerves; against the apoplexy, palsy, convulsions, megrim, vertigo, loss of memory, dimness of sight, melancholy, swooning fits and barrenness in women." It was given in canary, the syrup juice of black cherries, or in Florence wine. Country people have taken it in milk, or fair water, sweetened with sugar.

Lavender was used extensively in classical times by the Romans and Libyans, as a purification perfume for the bath. Greeks and Romans burned it as an incense offering to the Gods. Its bactericidal properties have been known for ages. It was certainly used in ancient Persia, Greece and Rome to disinfect hospitals and sick rooms.

Because of lavender's primarily balancing nature, it is of great value in helping people who are in an unbalanced emotional state, like hysteria, manic depression or just widely fluctuating moods.

Ancient druids carried lavender to aid in seeing ghosts, and to protect themselves against the "evil eye."

MUGWORT

Artemisia vulgaris

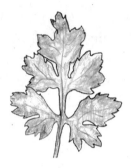

Mugwort is a symbol of health and hope. The plant grows freely in desolate, devastated places. The old town of Chernobyl was named for the plant. Mugwort thrives in overgrazed range lands of western North America, throughout the Russian Steppes, and in road cuts and landfills. It is nature's promise that life will spring anew.

Artemisia vulgaris can be recognized by its large dense stands of gray green scraggly bushes with tiny three-lobed leaves and coarse gray barked stems and trunks. The leaves are alternately five to seven lobes, with a silvery white color on the underside. The flowers are small ovoid, yellow to purplish, with numerous clusters blooming in July to August.

It is also known as wormwood, Altamisa, the herb of Saint John and black sage. Mugwort is under the influence of the planet Mars. It was mentioned in the Bible along with rue and was used by the Jews as one of the bitter herbs eaten during Passover.

In Europe, mugwort is known as croneswort, because it springs freely at the doorsteps of healers. Dr. John Hill extolled its virtues by saying, "Providence has placed it everywhere about our doors; so that reason and authority, as well as the notice of our senses, point it out for use." It is used to stimulate dreams and visions nearly everywhere it occurs.

All the Artemisias are insect repellents and likewise repugnant to bad spirits. In the Lakota tradition, it is believed it makes the bad spirits sick. They move away from it when it's burned. In ancient times, it was used as an antiseptic to counteract the poisons of hemlock, and some of the deadly Amanita mushrooms. Mrs. Greve, an Athapaskan healer, states that, "Mugwort and vinegar are an antidote to the mischief of mushrooms and henbane, and the biting of the seafish called Draco marinus or quaviver."

In the Middle Ages, the plant was known as *Cingulum Sancti Johannis*. It is believed that John the Baptist wore a girdle of it in the wilderness. On the longest day of the year, public bonfires were tended by young and old wreathed in garlands of mugwort and vervain. The people watched the flames through sprays of larkspur to improve their eyesight in the coming year. As they returned home, each one would throw his garland of herbs into the dying flames, asking the fire to burn away all of their bad luck.

Mugwort is a symbol of health and hope.

It was often claimed that divinational dreams could be improved by adding a half kilo of mugwort to one's pillow stuffing, and clairvoyant trances could be brought on by drinking mugwort tea. However, larger doses can be toxic.

Artemisia vulgaris has stimulant and slightly tonic properties. The volatile oil derived from the aerial parts of the plant have been used by women since ancient times to regulate menstruation, to prevent miscarriage, to speed up the birthing process and to expel the afterbirth. It also activates the digestive process and stimulates the liver.

As a nervine, mugwort is valued in palsy, epileptic and similar affections. Gerard, a German physician in the 1640s said, "Mugwort cureeth the shakings of the jooynts inclined to the Palsie." Another old writer affirmed that mugwort was good for the "quaking of the sinews."

The homeopathic physicians have used a tincture of the fresh root to treat catalepsy, chorea, convulsions, dysemenia, hydrocephalus, hysteria, somnambulism and worms.

In the folk medicine of Russia, the babushka uses the leaves, root and sometimes the whole plant when curing female illnesses. Some varieties include amenorrhoea, dysmenorrhoea, cramps, labor pains, as well as being used for convulsions, epilepsy, neurasthenia and other nervous disorders. It can be used for colds and stones including kidney, bladder and gall bladder. Roots and herbs are decocted for tubercular lungs. A decoction of the whole plant can be used for gastric conditions, nervousness, fright, convulsions, and overall female weakness.

Native American peoples use the leaves of mugwort medicinally in decoctions for colds, colic, bronchitis, rheumatism and fever.

OSHA

Ligusticum poteri

The incredible power of the osha plant is contained in its root. Large, dark brown and hairy, osha root convolutes and regrows in vast configurations. The energy of this North American herb is immediately apparent from its strong butterscotch-celery odor. The root is considered a talisman to many native peoples and is carried as a good luck charm.

There have been no successful efforts at cultivating osha plants.

Osha is the most widely used herbal medicine in the Southwest. Like other strong curing plants, osha has been used as a panacea, yet care must be taken in its identification. It resembles the poisonous hemlock and grows in a similar environment. It is found growing in the rugged western states, above 10,000 feet in altitude, in alpine clearings made by old burns and in logging cuts. Two of the best areas for harvesting osha are Taos, New Mexico, and in southern Colorado. Osha tenaciously refuses

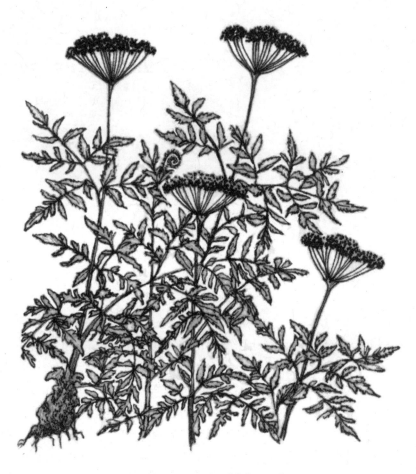

Osha is the most widely used
herbal medicine in the Southwest.

to be domesticated. There have been no successful efforts at cultivating osha plant.

The osha that appears above the ground is delicate and lovely. In
watery subalpine meadows, the osha plant creates a large and dis-
tinctive rosette at soil level. Its stalk is hollow like parsley, with large
basal leaves that may extend outward for up to two feet. At its
height of two feet, osha infloresces as a flat-topped umbrella, in
which the mature seeds can be found at the center.

Osha is a spicy, bitter, warm root that acts on the lungs and the stomach, producing sweats and fevers when necessary. It releases toxins, phlegm and gases from the body.

Wayfaring native peoples have carried osha root as a talisman to ward off rattlesnakes and witches' spells. Modern man is not aware of the power of his own mind in effecting others and influencing phenomena. Nor are we sufficiently trained in perceiving the influence of another's thoughts upon us. Our intellect has curtained the workings of magic in ordinary life. When the veil is opened, we see ways in which a plant that works to remove gross pathogenic factors also successfully dispels subtle negative energies.

Elders have always like to receive osha as a gift. The Navajo call it "deer eye," the Hopi call it "bear root," but osha is its Spanish name. White man has called osha "Porter's lovage," "'Colorado cough root," "bear medicine," and "Indian parsley." Nearly every Indian tribe in North America uses a species of Ligusticum, medicinally, ritually or symbolically. Osha is a plant associated with good luck and protection. It is revered by all traditional healers and medicine people living in the Southwest for its broadly effective and powerful healing abilities.

Used to treat colds, flu, fevers, cough, cold, phlegm diseases, indigestion, gas, delayed menses, and rheumatic complaints, osha has been called one of the most important herbs of the Rocky Mountains.

The Klamath Falls women burn osha root, using the smoke to perfume their hair and clothing. They also steam the root for facial treatments.

Apaches make a tea of osha for stomach ailments and people from the warm springs arch of Washington state chew the root to prevent colds.

PIÑON, NUT PINE

Pinus edulis

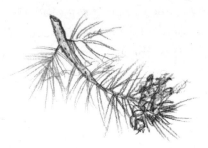

The Navajo people of North America have a variety of names for the different parts of the piñon tree (*Pinus edulis*). "Tcha"ol" or "Teestshiin" refer to the trunk of a dead tree. Piñon gum called "itjeeh." The nut is called "nictc'ii pina'a'." The wood is called "teetshiin," which if green, would be called "tch"ol." The needles are called "pi'iil." The native yellow ocher, used for dyes, is called "leetshoh" (earth, yellow).

Piñon pines are found in elevations around 5,000 feet. They form the timberline and cascade down below it. They live on arid, shallow, rocky soils of foothills, mesas and canyon walls. They occasionally grow in pure groves but usually are found in mixed stands of juniper, oak and yellow pine.

Piñon nuts are gathered in large quantities by Navajo women. They are either swept into piles and threshed, to remove the debris, or they are picked up off the ground by hand. Any of the excess nuts were sold or traded to the Zuni pueblos. The piñon nuts are roasted in pots or skillets, and sometimes mashed and made into a butter, similar to peanut butter. The nuts are crushed between two stones to remove the shell, and then made into a paste which is spread on hot corn cakes. The dried seeds of the piñon are made into necklaces, bracelets and anklets.

Piñon gum is used together with tallow and red clay to make a salve. The salve is prepared for use in open cuts and sores. The Navajo smeared the body of a dead person with piñon pitch before burying them. They wore the pitch under their eyes and on their forehead during the mourning period.

There are many ceremonials which include the use of the piñon. Indicated below are various ceremonies and the specific mode in which the piñon is offered. On the fourth day of the Night Chant ceremony, the Talking God carried a small sapling of piñon, almost entirely stripped of its branches. Piñon was used if the patient was male, and juniper was used if the patient was female. On the ninth day of the Night Chant, The Slayer of Alien Gods and The Child of the Water deposit their cigarettes, preferably in the shade of a piñon tree.

In the War Dance, the patient's body was painted with piñon and willow pitch. Dry piñon gum, together with the parts of several different birds, was burned as an incense. During the Mystery of the Night Chant initiates fumigated themselves with this incense. A corral was built for public exhibitions at the close of these ceremonials. It was built of juniper and piñon boughs, with an opening that faced to the east. Piñon needles were one of the ingredients used in making the medicine used in the War Dance. This remedy was taken internally. Piñon and juniper are also used in making the circle of branches for the Mountain Chant ceremony. During the last night of the Mountain Chant, the dancers carry bunches of piñon needles in each hand. Both hands are connected by wands extending out of the needles and creating an arch.

At the close of their ceremonies, members of the Zuni Order of Sword Swallowers, of the Great Fire Fraternity, will eat young buds of the piñon, if they desire female children. The young buds of the

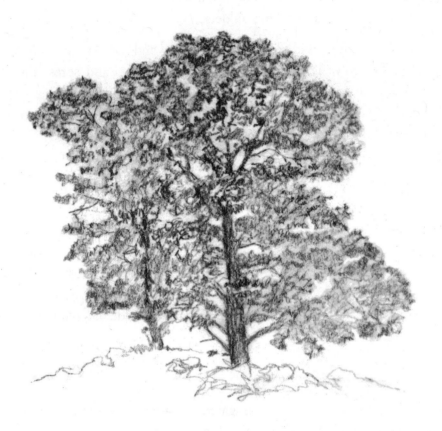

pine, called *Pinus brachyptera* or Yellow Pine, are eaten if they desire male children.

Medicinal Uses: Piñon is most useful after the feverish, infectious stage of a chest cold has passed. Piñon dredges hidden impurities from the depths of the system. It is used as a diuretic and expectorant. The pitch is rolled into a pellet the size of a berry, then chewed and swallowed. This is followed by a strong expectoration, which releases the lingering traces of disease. Like juniper berries, the piñon pitch expels urinary tract infections and should not be used if any inflammation is present.

The Navajo use the needles of the piñon tree for curing syphilis. The patient would chew the needles and swallow them. Next, they would drink a quantity of cold water. After drinking the water, they would run for about a mile, or until they would perspire profusely. The patient would return home and would be wrapped in a heavy blanket. Women afflicted with the same disease wrapped in blankets after taking the medicine, but did not participate in running.

At the War Dance ceremonies, if a person had fainted, the Navajo made a medicine from those plants which had been struck by lightning, and then a spruce and a piñon arrow would be shot over the body.

Piñon is also used by the Navajo as a dye. Sumac leaves are put in water and allowed to boil until the mixture becomes strong. While this is boiling, the ocher is powdered and roasted. Piñon gum is then added to the ocher and the whole of it is roasted again. As roasting proceeds, the gum melts and finally the mixture is reduced to a black powder. This is cooled and thrown into the sumac mixture, forming a rich blue-black fluid which is essentially an ink. When this process is finished wool is put in and allowed to boil until it is dyed to the correct shade. This same dye is also used to color leather and buckskin.

Hogans, both ordinary and ceremonial, are built of piñon logs, about eight to ten inches in diameter, and from ten to twelve feet long. Loom poles, beams, and uprights, for weaving rugs, are made of piñon wood. Ceremonial pokers, ceremonial wands, and various parts of the Navajo cradle, are also made of piñon wood because it is so easily carved. Piñon is used extensively for firewood. The best black sand for sand paintings is obtained from the charcoal of the piñon tree.

WHITE SAGE

Salvia apiana

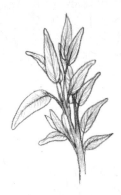

White sage grows along the sunny coastal alluvial washes of southern California, from Santa Barbara to the Baja Peninsula along the coast before the desert. White sage is an important member of the coastal sage scrub plants, growing two to three feet in height. It produces a flower spike that is light blue in color. The flower spikes produce a nectar and develop many seeds. The seeds have been important and potent food sources for wildlife and humans. The leaves vary from a matte green to a dull white, depending on the time of year. The leaves contain fragrant essential oils.

Today white sage is most popular for the sweet fragrance of its burning leaf. It is used to cleanse objects, places and people. The family Salvin, from the Latin, "salvia" (to heal), has many historical uses. Medicinally, white sage has been used as a tonic and as an antiseptic. Sage tea is said to promote a calming effect. Two leaves in a cup of hot water makes a healthful beverage, and the leaves may be chewed as a natural breath freshener.

Traditional elders say that before a person performs ceremony or is healed, they need to be cleansed of any bad feelings or negative thought. The cleansing can be done with sage, sweet grass or cedar. The smudging helps the healing come about in a very clear way, without any negative energy regarding the healer or the patient. The elders also say that one should enter into ceremony with a good heart.

The proper way to dispose of sage is to throw it eastward rather than burn it or put it down.

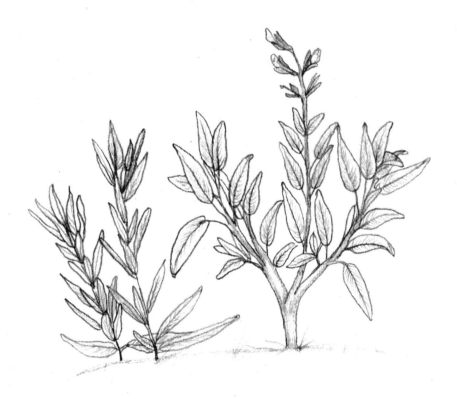

White sage flower spikes produce a nectar and develop many seeds.

White sage has come from relative obscurity twenty years ago to great popularity in recent years. People are attracted to its aroma and calming properties. The largest threat to its continued existence is loss of habitat through development of housing. Being part of the coastal scrub habitat there is a growing interest to preserve this unique plant community within private and public sectors.

According to Barbara Means Adams, wisdom receiver from the tribe of Black Elk, in her book *Prayers of Smoke*:

Sage, like sweet grass, is a symbol of cleanliness and purity. Tate, motion, son of the sky, gets his power from the sage plant.

Sage is a necessary part of every sacred ceremony. It is particularly important in the Sun Dance because the dancers chew it to alleviate their thirst. They wear crowns of sage. The silver-leaf sage plant is the incense of the seven sacred rituals. The leaf almost never dries out; it stays moist for a long time.

Another story about the origin of sage as a symbol involves the Little People again. The custom among them was to offer gifts each year to the White Buffalo Calf Woman. A poor girl, when her turn to give came, had nothing to offer. She plucked some weeds growing along her path and laid them at the White Buffalo Calf Woman's altar. So pure and fervent was her faith that the dry brown weeds turned to beautiful silver.

DESERT SAGE
Artemesia tridentata

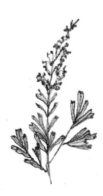

Desert sage brush covers much of the high plateau of the western states and is expanding its range. Sage brush bark provided fiber for footwear and clothing to the Fremont culture. Sage brush grows a protective cover for rabbits and small game, improving their habitat. With its many variations and names, big sage brush, mountain ball sage (*Artemesia frigida*), sweet sage (*Artemesia dracunculoderes*), black sage (*Artemesia nova*) as well as all its common tribal names, sage is a respected plant family.

Sage brush is the Nevada state flower and is used in its state Sun Dances as part of the dancer's costume and in many other dance regalia.

Sage can be used in numerous ways. It is traditionally used in ceremonies and included in medicine pouches and bundles. Sage is burned in smudging ceremonies to drive out bad spirits, feelings or influences. The leaves are valued for their aromatic properties and are used as a natural moth repellent. Native Americans of the Plains Nations cover the floor of their sweat lodges with sage. They will

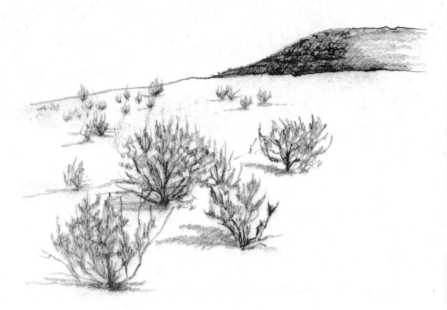

*Desert sage brush covers much of the high
plateau of the West.*

also breathe through a small bundle of sage and at times rub the
bundle on their bodies while in the sweat lodge. Some tribes commonly wrapped their pipes in sage before they bundled them up.
They believed that objects wrapped in sage were purified. Sage
wreaths are still placed around sundancers' heads, wrists and ankles
during the ceremony.

**Sage is a powerful tool
for well being.**

Traditional stories
and myths tell of the
power of sage, saying-
wherever sage is pres-
ent negative forces can-
not enter. In the Inipi

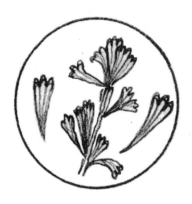

Desert sage is traditionally included in medicine pouches and bundles.

ceremony, a sprig of sage is worn behind the right ear to protect the participant and placate the Little People.

Hispanic people of the Southwest believe in sage as a powerful tool for well being and use sage tea to ward off coughs and colds. The fragrance alone is said to cure headaches and a poultice made of pounded leaves is said to be good for swellings and congestion. Known as chamiso hediondo, sage brush is used in stimulating sweats and breaking fevers. Extremely bitter, small quantities can aid in digestion. Externally, when mixed with oil or lard, it is used to inhibit fungus and bacteria.

Artemesia is named after the Greek goddess Artemesia (Diana), goddess of the hunt and the moon. To this day hunters rub themselves with sage to cover their scent. The mountains around Taos are memorable for the fragrance after rain covers the sage brush, filling the air with power.

SWEET GRASS

Hierochloe odorata

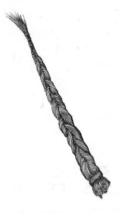

Sweet grass grows in the plains area of the United States and in Alberta, Canada. It is a tall, wide-bladed green grass with a reddish base. It is harvested when it reaches about fourteen inches in height. It smells pleasantly sweet when dried, and is traditionally braided together in long strands for storage and use.

Sweet grass can be burnt as a purifier similar to sage. It feels lighter than sage and is often burnt after using sage. It encourages positive vibrations to enter an area or room. Sweet grass is also used in sweat lodges. Clippings are placed on the hot rocks throughout the sweat. Participants can rub the leaves on their bodies while in the sweat.

An Oglala shaman describes the response of various spirits to the ceremonial smokes of sage and sweet grass:

> Inyan dwells in the stone. Tate dwells in the air. Okaga dwells in the south. Tatanka governs the love and hate of all men and all animals. I am a shaman. I am familiar

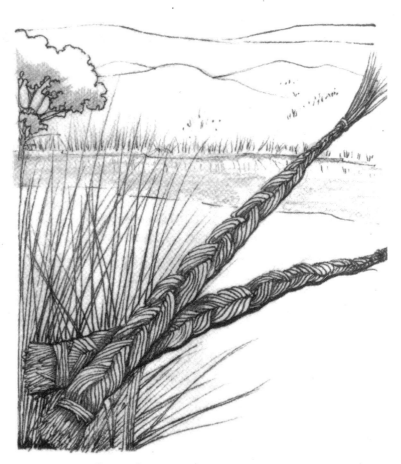

Sweet Grass encourages positive vibrations
to enter an area or room.

with these spirits. I am familiar with all spirits and the ghosts of dead men. They will do my bidding. When I make a medicine that is good, and when I make an incantation that pleases them, then, they will care for one whom I ask them to care for. This ceremony belongs in the tipi of Inyan. Tate and Okaga have taught it to the shamans.

Inyan wants one with a straight tongue. Tate wants one who is brave and cunning. Okaga wants one who has a good heart and is generous. Tatanka watches all Hunkyapi, and if they do wrong he informs all spirits of this and they punish such a one.

Okaga comes in the moon when the grass begins to grow. To the sweet grass he gives his spirit. His spirit is in the smoke of the sweet grass. Waza is the chief of the bad spirits. He brings cold and death. He hates Okaga, but he runs from the spirit of Okaga. The smoke of sweet grass and good song will drive the spirit of Waza away. Tate gives his spirit to the sage. The smoke of the sage is strong, and all evil spirits fear it. They will fly from it.

In Lakota ceremonials, sweet grass is used along with willow bark when choosing a shaman elder to instruct. A pipe is given to the chosen deputies of the apprentice and then sent to an elder, filled with dried willow bark and sweet grass. The ceremonial leader says:

Kola, go to his tipi. Take with you the pipe and this dried willow bark and this sweet grass and tell him I have chosen him to be my Ate. Tell him this because I honor him and wish him to teach me, so that I may become such a man as he is.

The same herbs are used by an old man or woman who are choosing a young person for apprenticeship. The one who proposes the relationships must provide the meeting place. They build the fire and furnish the willow bark and the sweet grass.

The ceremonial leader sits at the west, opposite the door, the students near the door, friends sit to the east, north and south side of the tipi. The student must fill the pipe, light it, and hand it to the maestro. The maestro smokes first and hands it to the friends. The teacher sprinkles the sweet grass on the fire. When they smoke the pipe for the second time, the teacher waves the pipe over the coals, in the smoke of the sweet grass saying, "Spirits, hear these my friends."

He then smokes the pipe, and hands it to one sitting in the east. The one in the east smokes and says, "Oh spirits of the east, we offer you this smoke.

The smoke of sweet grass is pleasant to the good spirits. They come to the smoke. They are pleased with one who makes this smoke.

Give us a bright day for this ceremony." He then gives it to the one in the north. That person smokes, and says, "Oh spirits of the Land of the Pines, give us a warm, pleasant day for the ceremony." He then smokes and hands it to the one who is in the south, who says, "Oh Spirit of the South, we offer you this smoke. Give us a generous day for the ceremony." He then smokes and hands it to the maestro. In this passage, a Lakota shaman describes the ways in which sage and sweet grass work in the spirit world.

Sage makes the bad spirits sick. They go away from it when it is burned. It does not make the good spirits sick. They will not leave when it is smoked. Sweet grass is pleasant to all the spirits. Good spirits like it. Bad spirits like it. All like it. The smoke of sweet grass is pleasant to the good spirits. They come to the smoke. They are pleased with one who makes this smoke. They will listen to what such a one asks. But the bad spirits come also to enjoy the smoke. So, sage must be burned to make them sick. Then, sweet grass to bring good spirits.

Barbara Means Adams, wisdom receiver from the tribe of Black Elk, tells of the origins of sweet grass in her book, *Prayers of Smoke*:

> Sweet grass, which Okaga, the south wind, introduced, is a part of almost all our rituals. Its life began when the world settled into the four seasons. It grows in the plains and mountains and can reach five feet in height. We cut it, braid it and dry it and then burn it to chase away evil spirits.
>
> The burning of sweet grass is a prayer, sent to heaven on the smoke. Wakan-Tanka is nature and understands fire and smoke much better than words. When I burn sweet grass, I don't mouth words. I just sit there and watch the smoke.

Sweet grass has universal use among American Indian tribes. It is for prayer and for cleansing. It can be a healing agent.

There are several other stories about the origin of sweet grass. One is that the Little People, who begin to appear regularly in stories from the second world, became so fascinated by their reflection in a pool that they pined away, leaving only a grass bearing their sweet fragrance, a memory of their vanity.

Another story is that sweet grass sprang up wherever the White Buffalo Calf Woman's tears fell as she changed from a red buffalo to yellow, to black, to white. White Buffalo Calf Woman is a major figure among the Sioux and appears in stories from the fourth world.

CEREMONIAL TOBACCO

Nicotine ssp.

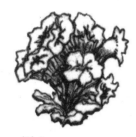

Tobacco as we commonly think of today is most often the commercial species *Nicotiana tabacum* grown for its large leaf. In the pre-Columbian Americas many species of *Nicotiana* were smoked, chewed, snuffed, insufflated, and used as enemas. Tobacco and water were offered to travelers when received in a home. Tobacco was offered to the gods to keep the world in balance and harmony.

Ceremonially, tobacco is smoked as a means of communication with spirit. The spirit world is asked for assistance and wisdom. The earthy substance, *Nicotiana*, is ignited, then transfigured into vapors and thus given in an honorable way to the astral land of the spirits. It is said that the ancestors remember the pleasure of smoking the leaves and the dried blossoms. So, they return to partake in the essence of the tobacco.

The people of North America all used tobacco like the communal meal. It tended to emphasize the inclusiveness of those partaking. The native tobacco was ceremonially planted and harvested by members of the tribes. For the people of the Blackfoot tribe, members gathered for a week at the sacred planting-grounds where elaborate ceremonies accompanied the sowing. John Hellson notes in *Ethnobotany of the Blackfoot Indians*:

> Between the period of planting and harvesting, taboos prevented anyone from visiting the plots, because the young plants were being tended by supernatural Small People, who did their gardening in return for offerings of miniature apparel, which had been left at the close of the planting ceremony.

In *The Smoking Gods: Tobacco in Maya Art History and Religion*, Francis Robicsek surveys the uses of tobacco by native peoples:

> The ancient Mayas and Aztecs were passionate smokers and so were their gods. Tobacco was given as an offering to the gods by the Seminoles, the Iroquois, some of the tribes east of the Rocky Mountains, and the nations of northwestern Venezuela. The Tupinamba of Brazil when smoking tobacco could go three or four days without eating anything else. Tobacco and tobacco smoke were used extensively in divination among the North and South American Indians and those of the Caribbean area. Among the Mazatecs, the curandero uses the paste of powdered tobacco and lime to render pregnant women invulnerable to witchcraft. The Yibaros of Rio Patesa and the Tucunas believed that tobacco augmented the magical properties of their bodies. The mountain tribes of Peru, the Jivaros and the Taparos, drank tobacco juice to prepare themselves for initiation into shamanhood. The Menominees buried the dead with a supply of tobacco to placate their gods.

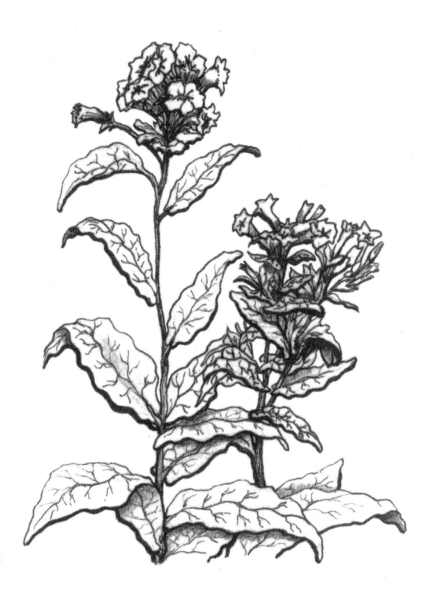

*Tobacco is smoked as a means of
communication with Spirit.*

The Tewas of San Ildefonso and the Omahas used tobacco to ensure the success of their hunt. The Tewas also used tobacco in their rain rituals to appease the gods of cloudbursts. Tobacco smoke was used in shamanistic divination by the Venezuelan tribes, the Florida Indians, the Guajiros of Colombia, several Caribbean groups, the Cumanos of the Orinoco River, the Warroas, the Puinavis, the Arawaks, the Caribs, and several other tribes.

Duran, a chronicler of the Aztec, noted that a magical ointment combining tobacco with oloiuhqui (morning-glory seeds) and ground venomous insects was called "the Divine Medicine."

This pitch also served a medicinal purpose: it was used to cure the sick and little children. Therefore, it was called the Divine Medicine, and people came from all parts to pay a visit to the dignitaries of the temple so as to be rubbed with the Divine Medicine. The People used the ointment to cure their ailments, since its properties are like those of picietal (tobacco) and oloiuhqui, which calm and soothe. Once it is applied as a plaster, it deadens pain; this it does by itself.

Tobacco was used extensively as a medicine outside Mesoamerica. The Roanoke Indians consumed tobacco to rid themselves of "bad humors." The Cherokees used tobacco leaves fried in butter to promote the healing of wounds. The Iroquois of New York placed wads of tobacco inside tooth cavities to ease pain. The Jivaro, Conibo, Campa, and Piro tribes of Peru cured headache and dysentery with tobacco. The Antives of Venezuela treated rheumatism with it.

Tobacco is found in plains and valley areas and is common along sandy washes. The various species are widespread along sandy washes throughout the United States. It likes dry stream beds, meadows, flats, flood plains and the desert. It has a knack for filling the empty nooks and crannies under abandoned highways and on the asphalt of trailer parks. It has been found growing upside down from the eroded lip of an arroyo.

To carry the tobacco blossoms, women of the plains tribes wore a basket made of the scrotum of a buffalo bull. This was hung down their back by a sarong strapped over the forehead or swung around on the breast. This would make it easy to drop the blossoms into it.

The blossoms and leaves were brought home to the lodge and spread out on a dry hide. They were placed in front of the sacred objects of the Big Birds' ceremony. The shrine might consist of two skulls and a sacred pipe, wrapped in a bundle. It was forbidden to walk between the fire and the shrine, as that would be a show of disrespect to the Gods.

When the sun was shining, the hide was moved to a place beneath the opening of the large smoke hole at the top of the lodge. There the sunbeam would fall on the blossoms and continue to dry them throughout the day.

The blossoms were then placed on a skin near the fire. A piece of buffalo fat was roasted over the fire at the end of a stick. Then the blossoms were touched here and there with the piece of buffalo fat.

Native American tobacco gardens were always cultivated by the elder men. A soft earthen plot, about eighteen by twenty feet in size, was made at the same time of year that the sunflower seed was planted. A big buffalo rib, sharpened on the edge, was used to work the soil and cultivate the tobacco. The elder would stoop down close to the ground and hold the buffalo rib in both hands with the edge pointed downward. Then with a song and a steady rhythmic motion, he would scrape the soil toward him, to loosen the earth for planting of the seeds.

The seeds are very small, brown, green and sticky and exceedingly numerous; as many as 1,000,000 may be produced by a single plant. These are laid down thickly, then covered lightly with soil. With the rain and warmth of the sun, the seeds sprout heartily. So many sprout at once they must be thinned out. They grow into a long scraggly bush composed of tall, wild branches and stems. The foliage is smooth, with a waxy grayish-blue bloom. The flowers are a pale, slightly yellow color. They grow completely tubular, until the end, where they flare out to form five tiny lobes.

The tobacco plant has long fibrous roots and an erect stem which is round, hairy and viscid. It branches near the top, which is from 3 to 6 feet high. The leaves are large and numerous, alternately attached to the stem. Stems form extended wings below the place of insertion, becoming egg-shaped at the broadest part. They are slightly viscid and hairy, pale-green in color, brittle and with a narcotic odor. They also have a bitter acrid taste.

The blossoms were considered the best part of the plant for smoking. They must be picked regularly, every fourth day after the season sets in. The blossoms are pinched off with the thumb nail. Once gathered, they are tipped slightly over the edge of the fire pit so that the heat from the fire can strike the blossoms. Now and then the blossoms are gently stirred with a little stick to oil the whole cluster equally.

When the grandfathers were ready to smoke these dried blossoms, they would draw them from the tobacco bag and chop them finely with a knife, one pipeful at a time. There are two ways to smoke tobacco. It is smoked for sacred reasons in ceremonials, and it is smoked socially, for pleasure.

Tobacco is also called tabacca, wild tobacco, punche, coyote tobacco, tree tobacco, Indian tobacco and mustard tree. It has various Indian names. Green tobacco is known as "Pwui-bamo" in Nevada. In Beatty, "Bahombe" means cured tobacco and may also mean cigarettes. The Owyhee people dry the whole plant and strip the slender leaves for their use, seeds and all. In Pyramid Lake, Paiute country, the whole plant is dried, diluted, and mixed with Bull Durham, Man-With-a-Coat-On, Prince Albert, or Toza for rolling tobacco.

Nicotianas leaves and blossoms can be cured, dried, and smoked. If used as a snuff it causes violent sneezing and a copious secretion of mucous. If chewed, it increases the flow of saliva by irritating the mucous membrane of the mouth. In large doses it produces nausea, vomiting, sweats and great muscular weakness.

By understanding the nature of tobacco's effect on the human body, we may come to a better understanding of the plant's relationship to spirit.

Medicinally, it is used to soothe overexcitement of the nervous system. It produces copious excretion of the urine by the kidneys. It assists in the removal of secretions from any air passages. It promotes vomiting, but should only used when other herbs for this purpose fail. When the smoke is injected into the rectum, or the leaf is rolled into a suppository, it has been beneficial in strangulated hernia. It will also produce evacuation of the bowels in case of obstinate constipation. It relieves spasmodic urethral stricture, hysterical convulsions, and spasms caused by lead poisoning.

Tobacco can also be used to relieve inflammation of the peritoneum. It moderates reaction in tetanus and dispels timpanists. A wet tobacco leaf, applied to piles, is a certain cure. The tobacco juice cures facial neuralgia if rubbed along the tracks of the affected nerve. The leaves, in combination with the leaves of belladonna or stramonium, make an excellent application for obstinate ulcers, painful tremors, and spasmodic afflictions.

Offerings of Tobacco, Sweat Lodge Speech/Winnebago Clan Ceremonial from the Winnebago Tribe

I greet you; I greet you all, war bundle owners. My grandparents, especially my grandfather had concentrated their minds upon this for me. The fireplace with which they blessed my grandfather, that I am going to ask for myself. However weakly I may wobble about, my elders will aid me. I am now going to pour a little tobacco and offer, my elders, whatever feast I am able to. War bundle owners, I send forth my greetings to you. War bundle owners, I greet you. You elders, I am about to pour tobacco for them.

Hearken, Earthmaker, our father, I am about to offer you a handful of tobacco. My ancestor Jobenangiwingkha concentrated his mind upon you. The fireplaces with which you blessed him; the small amount of life you granted to him; all, four times the blessings you bestowed upon my ancestor, that I ask of you directly. Also that I may have no trouble.

To you, who live in the west, our grandfather, chief of the Thunderbirds, a handful of tobacco I am about to offer you. My grandfather, Jobenangiwingkha, you strengthened. The food, the deer-couple you gave him for his fireplaces, that I ask of you directly. May it be a fact that you accept this tobacco from me and may I not meet with troubles.

You also, Great Black Hawk of the North, blessed my grandfather. Whatever food you blessed him with that I ask of you directly. Tobacco I am about to pour for you that you may smoke it. May troubles not come upon me; that I ask of you directly. Also that I may have no trouble.

To you, who live in the west, our grandfather, chief of the Thunderbirds, a handful of tobacco I am about to offer you. My grandfather, Jobenangiwingkha, you strengthened. The food, the deer-couple you gave him for his fireplaces, that I ask of you directly. May it be a fact that you accept this tobacco from me and may I not meet with troubles.

You also, Great Black Hawk, blessed my grandfather. Whatever food you blessed him with that I ask of you directly. Tobacco I am about to pour for you that you may smoke it. May troubles not come upon me; that I ask.

You on the other side, who live in the east, who walk in darkness, tobacco I am about to offer you to smoke. Whatever you blessed my ancestor with, whatever fire-places you blessed him with, those I ask of you. If you smoke this tobacco, never will I be a weakling.

You who live in the south, you who look like a man, who art invulnerable; who on one side of your body present death and on the other life, Disease Giver, as they call you. My ancestor in the daytime, in broad daylight, did you bless. With food you blessed him. You told him that he would never fail in anything. You told him that you would avoid his home. You placed animals in front of him that he should not be troubled about obtaining them. An offering of tobacco I make to you that you may smoke it and that I may not be troubled by anything.

To you, Light-Wanderer, an offering of tobacco I make. May it be my good fortune that you accept it. Whatever fireplaces you blessed him with, those I ask of you directly. May I not be troubled by anything in life.

You also, Grandmother Moon, blessed my ancestor with food. With whatever you blessed him, that I ask of you now directly. An offering of tobacco I am about to make for you now, so that by reason of it I may never become a weakling.

To you, too, South Wind, I offer a handful of tobacco, that you may smoke it. May it so happen that you accept it and that I am spared troubles. With whatsoever you blessed my ancestor, that I ask of you.

For you likewise, Grandmother Earth, will I pour tobacco. With whatever blessings you blessed my grandfather, those I ask of you. May I in that way never become a weakling.

To you, a pair of Eagles, my ancestor prayed. The blessings you bestowed upon him, those I ask of you. I am about to pour a handful of tobacco for you. May you accept it and ward off trouble from me.

Hearken, all you spirits to whom my ancestor prayed; to all of you, I offer tobacco. My ancestor Jobenangiwingkha gave a feast to all those who had blessed him, and we are repeating this now. However, as it is about time to proceed to the next part we will ask you once again to bestow upon us all the blessings you gave our ancestor. That we may not become weaklings, I ask of you. I greet you all.

The Pipe

The word "tobacco" came from a peculiar instrument used for inhaling its smoke by the inhabitants of Hispaniola, San Domingo. The instrument, described by Oviedo, consisted of a small hollow wooden tube, shaped like a "Y," the two points of which were inserted in the nose of the smoker, the other end was held into the smoke of burning tobacco, and thus the fumes could be inhaled. The apparatus the natives called "tabaco."

The pipe of the Native Americans has a different form. In order to make a pipe, the Plains Indian novice would go to a great pipe-stone quarry, like those common to Minnesota. There, he would roam the dark red terrain, searching for a stone shaped like the letter "L." If the pipestone was newly mined, it would be soft enough to form with the hands, into an eight inch length so the pipe bowl would be as large as a man's thumb.

The pipe-stem was made of golden sumac, which grew close by the pipestone quarry. The sumac was gathered in the spring when the sap was up, in the large pith. The piece of sumac was put in a can of oil or bear grease. A piece of bear meat or fish was put out where the blow flies could work on it. When large maggots were on the meat, the oil-softened pith of the sumac was brought in. The maggots were sealed up in the stem and would eat their way through, boring a perfect hole. On either side of this hole, column holes were made. These were made in sets of two, about six sets to the middle of the stem. Through these holes buckskin strings were inserted and on them treasures of old Hudson Bay beads, preferably blue, were tied. Sometimes, abalone shell pendants would be hung with brightly colored bird feathers to attract spirit. Eagle down was put on, so that the pipe could "float."

Prayer to the Ghost with Tobacco

Here it is, the tobacco. I am certain that you,
    O ghost, are not very far away, that in fact
    you are standing right in back of me, waiting
    for me to reach you the pipe and tobacco,
    that you might take it along with you, that like
    wise you are waiting for your food to take on
    your journey. However, four nights you will have
    to remain here.
Now here are these things, and in return we ask you
    to act as mediator (between the spirits and us).
    You have made us long for you, and therefore
    see to it that all those things that belonged to
    you and that you would have enjoyed had you
    lived longer—victories on the warpath,
    earthly possessions and life—that all these things
    you leave behind for us to enjoy.
This you must ask for us as you travel along.
This also I ask of you:
    do not cause us to follow you soon;
    do not cause your brothers any fear.
I have now lit the pipe for you.

Winnebago

To Make Tobacco When They Are Hurting Somewhere

Listen! You and I have just come together
　　to unite our efforts.
You and I are Great Wizards.
You and I are to fail in nothing.
Each of the Seven Clan Districts is not to climb
　　over you and me!
Listen! Brown Whirlwind itself!
You and I have just come together to unite our efforts.
You and I are Great Wizards.
You and I are to fail in nothing.
Each of the Seven Clan Districts is not to climb
　　over you and me!

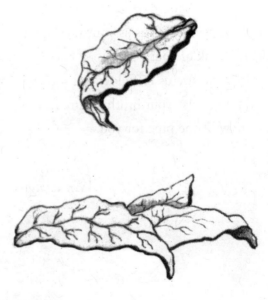

RED WILLOW BARK
RED OSHER DOGWOOD

Cornus sericea

The dogwood family has evolved along a distinct path. It is considered a relative of the four winds. Red willow bark (red osher dogwood) and the cottonwoods stand on their own, being especially adapted to having the winds sow their seeds. Its apparent kinship to the spirits of the air give these trees their sacred qualities. American Indians use the gift of dogwood's bark for reducing fevers. The bark and branches of red willow are used to make wands and prayer sticks in ceremony, seem conducive to communication through the air.

Red willow (red osher dogwood) changes, mutates, and adapts from stream to stream. As we see in the case of other trees and plants, the best medicine spirit is always mutable and versatile, while imparting its strength. We find thickets of red willow bark stabilizing sandy shores of

The best medicine spirit is always mutable and versatile

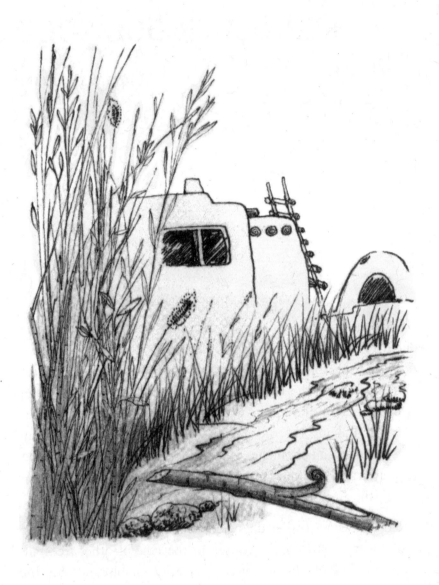

Red willow . . . relative of the four winds.

washes, streams and water impoundments up to elevations of about 7,000 feet. It is found growing in communities with the Fremont cottonwood, Russian olive, tamarisk, and goodding willow.

Dogwood is employed in many ways. Most of the dogwoods have been used for their pain-relieving and fever-lowering properties. The fresh bark contains salicin, which probably decomposes into salicyclic acid in the human system. Aspirin, a well-known drug taken for its analgesic and febrifuge effects, is chemically related to salicylic acid.

The Natchez people prepared their fever remedies from the bark of the red willow, while the Alabama and Creek Indians plunged into willow root steam baths for the same purpose. The use of dogwood is also reported among the Pima of Arizona, the Houma of Mississippi, the Mohegans of Connecticut, the Penobscots of Maine, the Montagnais of southeastern Canada, and many other American tribes. Hopi and Navajo clans use willow to make prayer sticks and amulets.

In most cases the ceremonial use of red willow bark is wind related, with a secondary relationship to water. Heald sticks used in weaving, praryer sticks, prayer stick foundations, permanent carrying baskets, cradle canopies and plumed wands are all made of willow. Water bottles were made or sewed with it. A braided willow strap was worn across the forehead and used to support the water bottle. Lances were formerly made of red willow hardened by pounding it with a stone. Arrow shafts were made of red willow.

In the Navajo Mountain Chant ceremony, red willow sticks are gathered to make the emblem of the concentration of the four winds. A square was made with these sticks, leaving the ends projecting at the corners. The square is then placed over the invalid's head. For the rite of charcoal painting in Night Chant, a quantity of willow sticks, together with several pieces of pine bark, are burned into charcoal. The ashes of two different kinds of weeds, together with the ashes of two small feathers, are then added to the fat of a goat, mountain sheep or another animal and made into balls. Then the salve is daubed on appropriate parts of the body. The talisman used in the Night Chant consists of four sticks of peeled red willow bark.

In the Hopi tradition, from the villages of the East Mesa in the province of Tusayan, prayer sticks are made by a crowd of women members inside the kiva. They are also called Willow Wands. Many of the prayer sticks are funerary in character. Their occurrence in burials is evidence of this. Votive prayer sticks to the Death God Masauwuh, in the Snake Drama at Walpi, are also made from the branches of red willow.

Medicinal uses: Red willow bark, (red osher dogwood) is useful for headache, fevers, neuralgia, and hay fever. Its uses are many, but most specifically in the reduction of inflammations of joints and membranes.

YERBA SANTA

Eriodictyon californicus

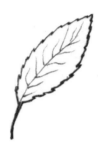

Yerba santa is also called "Portable Temple" (Matthew Wood), because it will drive out the negative influences in an environment and restore a guarded boundary of protection. The leaves may be scattered around the bed of someone with a degenerative disease. Because of these qualities, yerba santa may be burned as incense to create a sanctuary conducive for healing.

Also known as mountain balm, bear's weed, consumptive's weed, tarweed and gum bush, this evergreen shrub is two to four feet high, wooly-wooly or shiny-wooley species, with furry lanced leaves and tubular purple or blue flowers in terminal clusters of six to ten. Yerba santa grows in clumps on dry hills in California, northern Mexico and Arizona.

Yerba santa is a member of the water leaf family (Eriodictyon). Its name was given by the Spanish priests, who became aware of this corrective substance through the Native Americans. They boiled the fresh or dried leaves for colds, coughs, sore throat, catarrh or stomach aches. Edward Palmer wrote in 1978, that it was "a great

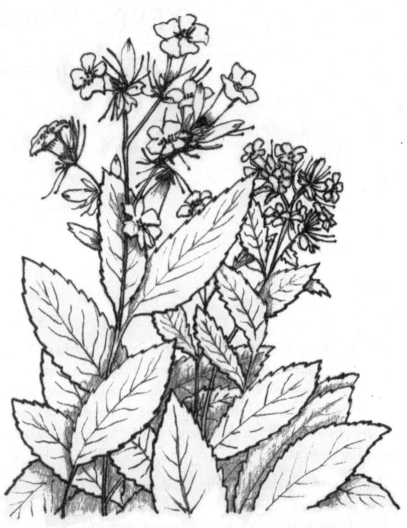

Yerba Santa will drive out the negative influences in an environment and restore a guarded boundary of protection.

medicine among the Indians of southern Utah, Arizona and California." It is taken internally for rheumatism and partial paralysis, or applied externally. For lung infections the dry leaves were chewed or smoked, or taken as a tea.

Yerba santa is used as an expectorant in the treatment of chronic pulmonary infections. The festering or degenerate tissue is expelled from the depths to the surface. The protective membranes are revived and toned. According to the doctrines of homeopathy, a pathology must be ultimated, must come into full bloom at the surface of the organism, to be cleared away. The active ingredients of yerba santa, its resins and phenols, are strongest right after blooming. When smoked or taken internally as a tea, hidden weaknesses, untruths, fears and disease are forced to the surface of the body, where they may quickly amplify and eventually disappear.

Degenerative diseases, which open the vital organs to predatory influences are countered by yerba santa which reestablishes the boundary conditions of protection. The membranes that guard the vital organs are toned; it has long been used as a woundwort or herbal bandage for broken skin. The Renaissance Doctrine of Signatures was the physicians' way of reading the forms of the botanical environment for clues as to their medicinal relationship to the forms of the anatomy of the human organism. The bronchial veins on the underside of yerba santa bring to mind similar branching systems that line the lungs and bronchial of air breathing creatures.

The mucilaginous or glutinous resin that covers the upper side of the plant is like a mucous membrane. This is an indicator that its sphere of action is in the lungs and throat. The smooth, furry upper surface can be likened to the pleural linings. It is in the realm of internal body linings in which yerba santa has its special application. It is this guarding quality, this tendency to restore healthy boundary conditions, that leads healers to use yerba santa to clear psychic toxins from a room.

Yerba santa is known to physicians as a leading agent for all respiratory conditions and has a reputation for healing hemorrhoids when other sources fail. It became an official pharmaceutical, marketed by Parke Davis and Company in 1894.

Prayer

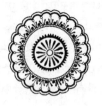

Owl!

I have made your sacrifice.

I have prepared a smoke for you.

My feet restore for me.

My legs restore for me.

My body restore for me.

My mind restore for me.

My voice restore for me.

Today take out your spell form me.

Today your spell for me is removed.

Away from me you have taken it.

Far off from me it is taken.

Far off you have done it.

Today I shall recover.

Today for me it is taken off.

Today my interior shall become cool.

My interior feeling cold, I shall go forth.

My interior feeling cold, may I walk.

No longer sore, may I walk.

Impervious to pain, may I walk.

Feeling light within, may I walk.

With lively feelings, may I walk.
Happily may I walk.
Happily abundant dark clouds I desire.
Happily abundant showers I desire.
Happily abundant vegetation I desire.
Happily abundant pollen I desire.
Happily abundant dew I desire.
Happily may I walk.
May it be happy before me.
May it be happy behind me.
May it be happy below me.
May it be happy above me.
With it happy all around me, may I walk.
It is finished in beauty.
It is finished in beauty.

Navajo

Bibliography

This book represents a synthesis of thoughts, words and research of herbalists, ethnographers, and authors who dedicated many years of investigation into the uses of sacred herbs for ceremonial purposes. These master works include the following:

Adams, Barbara Means. *Prayers of Smoke*, Celestial Arts, Berkeley, Calif., 1990.

Bierhorst, John. *In the Trail of the Wind: American Indian Poems and Ritual Orations*, Farrar, Straus & Giroux, New York, N.Y., 1971.

Brown, Joseph Epes. *The Sacred Pipe, Black Elk's Account of the Seven Rites of the Oglala Sioux*, University of Oklahoma Press, Norman, Okla.

Bunzel, Ruth. *Zuni Ceremonialism*, University of New Mexico Press, Albuquerque, N.Mex., 1992.

Boas, Franz. *The Ethnology of the Kwakiutl, Contributions to Anthropology Series*, Vol. 3, Columbia University, 1977.

Castleman, Michael. *The Healing Herbs: The Ultimate Guide to the Curative Power of Nature's Medicines*, Rodale Press, Emmaus, Pa., 1991.

Coggins, K. *Alternative Pathways to Healing: The Recovery Medicine Wheel*, Health Communication, Deerfield Beach, Fla., 1990.

Cunninghman, Scott. *Encyclopedia of Magical Herbs*, Llewellyn Publications, St. Paul, Minn., 1992.

Cunningham Scott. *Magical Herbalism, Llewellyn's Practical Magick Series*, Llewellyn Publications, St. Paul, Minn., 1982.

Davis, Patricia. *Aromatherapy an A-Z*, Beekman Publications, Woodstock, N.Y., 1991.

Dawson, Adele G. *Herbs, Partners with Life*, S. Greene Press, Brattleboro, Vt., 1980.

Dooling, D.M. and Paul Jordan Smith. editors. *I Become Part of It: Sacred Dimensions in Native American Life*, Parabola Books, N.Y., 1989.

Foster, Steven and Meredith Little. *The Roaring of The Sacred River, A Sun Bear Book*, Prentice Hall Press, N.Y., 1989.

Gilbert L. Wilson. *Buffalo Bird Woman's Garden, Agriculture of the Hidatsa Indians*, Minnesota Historical Society Press, St. Paul, Minn., 1987.

Harrington, H.D. *Edible Native Plants of the Rocky Mountains*, The University of New Mexico Press, Albuquerque, N.Mex., 1967.

Hausman, Gerald. *Turtle Island Alphabet: a Lexicon of Native American Life*, Parabola Books, N.Y., 1989.

Hellson, John. *Ethnobotany of the Blackfoot Indians*.

Herbalgram, The Journal of the American Botanical Council and the Herb Research Foundation, Austin, Tex.

Hutchens, Alma R. *A Handbook of Native American Herbs*, Shambhala Press, Boston, Mass. and London, England, 1992.

Hutchens, Alma R. *Indian Herbology of North America*, Shambhala Publications, Inc., Boston, Mass., 1973.

Hungry Wolf, Adolf. *A Good Medicine Collection*, The Book Publishing Co., Summertown, Tenn., 1990.

Junemann, Monika. *Enchanting Scents*, Lotus Light Books, 1998.

Klein, B. *Reference Encyclopedia of the American Indian*, Todd Publications, N.Y., 1986.

Liebert, Robert. *Osage Life and Legends: Earth People. Sky People.* Naturegraph, Happy Camp, Calif., 1987.

Mabey, Richard. *The New Age Herbal*, Guild Publishing, London, England, 1985.

Mayes, Vernon O. and Barbara Bayless Lacey. *Nanise, A Navajo Herbal*, Navajo Community College Press, Tsaile, Ariz., 1989.

Medicine Hawk. *American Indian Ceremonies: A Practical Wookbook and Study Guide to the Medicine Path*, Global Communications, Inner Light, N.Y., 1992.

Moore, Michael. *Medicinal Plants of The Desert and Canyon West*, The Museum of New Mexico Press, Santa Fe, N.Mex., 1977.

Moore, Michael. *Medicinal Plants of The Mountain West* , The Museum of New Mexico Press, Santa Fe, N.Mex., 1979.

Moore, Michael. *Los Remedios, Traditional Herbal Remedies of The Southwest*, Red Crane Books, Santa Fe, N.Mex., 1990.

Mowrey, Daniel B. *The Scientific Validation of Herbal Medicine*, Keats Publishing Inc., New Canaan, Conn., 1986.

Murphy, Edith Van Allen. *Indian Uses of Native Plants*, Mendocino County Historical Society, Fort Bragg, Calif., 1959.

Radin, Paul. *Crashing Thunder, The Autobiography of An American Indian.* D. Appleton Co., N.Y., 1926.

Robicsek, Francis. *The Smoking Gods: Tobacco in Maya Art History and Religion*, University of Oklahoma Press, Norman, Okla., 1978.

Tedlock, Dennis. *The Popul Vuh, with commentary based on the ancient knowledge of the Quiche Maya.*

Tierra, Michael. *Planetary Herbology*, Lotus Press, Santa Fe, N.Mex., 1979.

Van Gennep, Arnold. *The Rites Of Passage*, University of Chicago Press, Chicago, Ill., 1960.

Vecsey, Christopher. *Imagine Ourselves Richly, Mythic Narratives of North American Indians*, Harper Collins Paperback, New York, N.Y., 1991.

Vogel, Virgil J. *American Indian Medicine, The Civilization of The American Indian Series*, University of Oklahoma Press, London, 1970.

Walker, Barbara G. *A Woman's Dictionary of Symbols and Sacred Objects*, Harper & Row, San Francisco, Calif., 1988.

Walker, James R. *Lakota Belief and Ritual*, Bison Books, University of Nebraska Press, Nebr., 1991.

Walking Nighbear & Padilla, Stan. *Song of The Seven Herbs*, The Book Publishing Company, Summertown, Tenn., 1987.

Weiner, Michael. *Earth Medicine, Earth Food*, Macmillan, New York, N.Y., 1972.

Wilbert, Johannes. *Tobacco and Shamanism in South America*, Yale University Press, New Haven, Conn., 1987.

Wilson, Maggie. "Naming Beverly's Baby," *Native People's Magazine*, vol. 1, #1, pp. 2-5, 1990.

Ywahoo, Dhyani. *Voices of Our Ancestors*, Shambhala Press, Boston, Mass., 1987.

Index

red osher dogwood *see* red willow
red willow 8, 9, 48, 94, 111-114
  Alabama 113
  Blackfoot 30
  Creek 113
  Crying for a Vision 27, 28
  description 111, 113
  Hopi 113, 114
  Lakota 94
  medicinal uses 8, 9, 113, 114
  Natchez 113
  Navajo 113-114
  Night Chant 113-114
  Oglala Sioux 30
  Pima 113
  Sun Dance ceremony 48
  Sweat Lodge ceremony 29-30
  totem 48
  War Dance 83
Releasing of the Soul Rite 41, 43, 44
rheumatism 58, 61, 70, 78, 81, 100, 117
Rio Patesa 98
rites of passage 24
ritual
  Native American forms 14, 100
  personal 14-15
  purifying ignorance 15
  to enact 8
  to remember 7
Roanoke Indians 100
Rocky Mountains 55, 60, 81, 98
sacred
  beings 11, 42
  buckskin 40
  bundle 37
  circle 30
  clowns 47, 48
  dance 32
  days 33, 41, 42
  hoop 33, 37, 40
  manner 33, 36, 38
  objects 33, 37, 40-44, 101
  paths 33, 36, 40, 41, 44
  pipe 41, 42, 43, 101
  place 39, 62
  planting-grounds 98
sacred plants 8, 9, 11, 14, 18, 32,
  47, 48, 49, 62, 68, 88, 102, 111
sacred woman 38, 39
sage 23-24, 28, 31, 33, 48, 49, 87-92
  Blackfoot use 34

sage *continued*
  burning of 20, 26-27, 37, 49,
    61, 89, 95, 96
  chewed in sweat lodge 30
  cleansing 87
  coming of age ceremony 25
  Crying for a Vision 27-29
  description 86
  disposing of 87
  Keeping of the Soul Rite 37
  Lakota use 95
  Little People 88, 91
  medicinal use 86, 91
  shamans use 94
  Sun Dance 33-34, 88, 90
  Sweat Lodge 29-32, 61, 90
salicin 113
salicinin 9
salicylic acid 113
Salvia apiana 86
San Ildefonso Pueblo 100
sand paintings 85
savin 58, 61
scurvy 58, 61
Seminoles 98
shaman 92, 93, 94, 95, 98, 100
Shoshone 70
Shungopavi 21
Sioux 24, 25, 27, 30, 96
smallpox 70
smudging 49, 50, 87, 89
somnambulism 78
Sonora Desert 65
sore throat 115
soul bundle 37
soul keeper 37, 41
soul sustenance 11
space
  extraordinary 14, 15, 18
  ordinary 8, 14, 15, 18
  sacred 7, 8, 16
spirit world 95, 97
spiritual
  essence 9
  event 7
  foundations 14
  intention 9-10
  love 74
  nature 7
  practices 15
  root 49
stomach aches 71, 75, 81, 115

stramonium 103
sumac 85, 107, 108
Sun Dance 24, 27, 30-34, 88, 89, 90
sunflower 101
Sweat Lodge 24-26, 29-32, 58, 61,
    71, 90, 92, 104
sweet grass 23-24, 48-49, 87-88,
    92, 94-96
    burning of 20, 26-27, 31, 37, 49,
        92, 95
    coming of age ceremony 25
    Crying for a Vision 27, 29
    Keeping of the Soul Rite 37, 40
    Releasing of the Soul Rite 44
    Sweat Lodge ceremony 29-32
syphilis 85
talisman 79, 81, 114
talking circle 38
Talking God 83
tannic acid 61
Taos 79, 91
Taparos 98
tarweed 115
Tatanka 92, 94
Tate 92, 93, 94
tetanus 103
Tewa Indians 68, 100
Thunderbeing 42, 48, 62
Thunderbirds 51, 104, 105
time
    extraordinary 14, 15, 18
    ordinary 7, 8, 14, 15, 18
    sacred 7, 8, 17
    spirit in 10
tobacco 11, 27, 49, 51, 52, 97-110
    Arawaks 100
    Aztecs 98, 100
    Blackfoot 29, 97
    bundle 28
    Caribs 100
    Cherokee 20, 100
    communion 97
    Crying for a Vision ceremony 27
    description 100, 101, 102
    divination 98, 100
    gardens 101
    Guajiros 100
    Iroquois 98
    Keeping of the Soul 37-38
    Maya 98
    medicinal uses 100, 103

tobacco *continued*
    offerings 20, 27, 28, 31, 51-52,
        97-98, 104-106
    Oglala Sioux 24, 28
    Paiutes 103
    paste 98
    Releasing of the Soul Rite 42
    Seminoles 98
    Spirit communication 97
    Sun Dance 33
    Sweat Lodge 29-32, 104-105
    Tewas 100
    Tupinamba 98
    Winnebago 104, 109
Tsalagi 20, 47
Tucunas 98
Tupinamba 98
Two-Hearts 22
ulcers 103
urinary tract infections 84
vermifuge 75
vervain 77
vision fasting 26
vision quest 26, 27, 29
Wakan-Tanka 32-44, 96
wands 30, 83, 85, 111, 113, 114
war bonnet 27
war bundle 104
War Dance 83, 85
Warroas 100
warts 58, 61
White Buffalo Calf Woman 88, 96
white sage 86-88
White Swan 43
willow, red *see* red willow
Winnebago 51, 104, 109
witchcraft 12, 81, 98
Wiwanyag Wachipi 24, 32
worms 78
wormwood 76
Wounded Knee 37
yerba santa 115-118
    ceremonial use 116, 18
    description 115, 117
    incense 115
    medicinal uses 115, 117, 118
Yibaros 98
Ywahoo, Dhyani 15, 20, 44, 47
Zuni 5, 57, 82, 83

About the Author

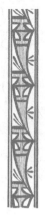

Alfred Savinelli has wildcrafted plants for the past twenty years in the Americas (North, South, and Central). He has primarily gathered plants for ceremonial and ritual use by Native People. His efforts have grown to include a network of Native People who gather plants in a sacred and ecological manner.

Promoting health and well-being through spiritual harmony, Alfred is an active defender of plant rights and indigenous wisdom. He is currently working with Native Scents, Inc. in Taos, New Mexico, which produces a wide range of aromatic herbal products and related items.

About *Plants of Power*, Alfred Savinelli says, "Much of the insightful information in this book comes from talking with thousands of people about these plants and finding new bits of forgotten wisdom. This is a process that will continue through my lifetime of discovery and service."

All comments, inquiries and suggestions may be sent in care of Native Scents, Inc., Box 5639, Taos, NM 87571

Taos, New Mexico
November, 2001